# The Healing Power of FLAX

by Herb Joiner-Bey, N.D.

Disclaimer: The author provides the information in this book
to acquaint health care professionals and the public
with the health benefits of flaxseed for educational purposes
only. The information is derived from a judicious synthesis of
traditional and clinical experience and verified by scientific
research. It is intended for use by professionals seeking to
apply the principles of natural medicine to the needs of their
patients or by patients under the direct supervision and guid-
ance of such professionals. It is not intended as a means for
patients to self-diagnose and/or self-medicate without the
sound judgment and seasoned counsel of a well-informed
health care provider. We strongly urge the patient to consult
an appropriately educated health care provider before making
any changes to health maintenance or therapeutic regimens.

Book design by Bonnie Lambert

ISBN 1-893910-32-6
Second printing
Printed in the United States
Published by Freedom Press
1801 Chart Trail
Topanga, CA 90290
Bulk Orders Available: (800) 959-9797
E-mail: info@freedompressonline.com

# Acknowledgements

The author wishes to acknowledge with great appreciation the research and writings of Jade Beutler, of Barlean's Organic Oils, whose work has served as the basis and infrastructure for this book. Moreover, I acknowledge Jade's asking me to participate in this worthwhile project. Thank you, Jade, for the opportunity to be of service.

Next, I must acknowledge Jim Springer, also of Barlean's, whose diplomatic liaison efforts moved this endeavor beyond the breakdowns and obstacles that inevitably arise during the manifestation of bold possibilities. Of course, I also wish to thank my editors and designers at Freedom Press: Cassandra Glickman, Marcy Crawford, Bonnie Lambert and John Odam.

I would also like to express my gratitude to David Steinman, the vision and dynamism behind Freedom Press, for his hard work in assembling the initial draft of this book and for attending to the details of editing and publishing with professionalism and patience. Thank you, David, for a great learning experience.

I also wish to thank Michael Minarsich and Michael Loes, M.D., M.D.(H.), for their great support and commitment to excellence in all things. I especially am thankful that Michael Minarsich had the great foresight to partner with Bruce Barlean of Barlean's to make the finest, organic highest lignan flaxseed oil available throughout the world. Thanks, Mike.

# Contents

# Foreword

The miracles of flax began trickling into American awareness soon after Dr. Johanna Budwig presented her research findings. The year was 1959. The place was Zurich, Switzerland. Dr. Budwig concluded that essential fatty acids—especially omega-3—played a significant role in cancer. She determined that early cancer cells had fat abnormalities. Taking omega 3 fatty acids prevented the development of these abnormal cells. While it would take years for this seminal research to be appreciated, the latchkey had been sprung.

Let's fast forward to 1986. In America, flaxseed oil was known as "linseed oil." Though its health-enhancing properties had continued to get international press, the federal Food and Drug Administration (FDA) prohibited flax from being imported into the U.S. The beneficial health claims made about flaxseed oil were dismissed. Americans were unable to find or purchase reliable, cold-pressed, organic flaxseed oil even though elsewhere in the world the health buzz was already spreading.

In 1986, Michael Minarsich and Bruce Barlean, a salmon fisherman in northern Washington near the Canadian border, also saw this potential need. Both men had concluded that although salmon was a great source of omega 3, ocean salmon was scant at times and was not enough of a source to meet this growing demand. The superior benefit of flax oil and its lignans could be clearly identified. Getting a supply of flax for Americans became *a timely and important task*. Both men knew that where there is a resolved will, there is a definitive way. The challenge was to somehow open the closed importation door.

Through a series of creative lobbying and legal strategies, the two men succeeded in bringing flax to America. This successful maneuver working with the system for the public benefit *allowed the hats to tip and the documents to be signed clearing the way for flax*.

The lesson learned was an old one from the adage, "Give the opportunity for your enemy to become your friend." This has happened; today, the FDA allows health claims to be made for flax. With creative problem-solving, Mr. Minarsich and Mr. Barlean scored a victory. The result is an open border and a readily available pure product that enhances the healing response. Indeed, both men work together to this day to supply the world with what many connoisseurs and health conscious consumers say is the most flavorful and lignan rich flax oil in the world today.

On a personal note, I am an aging athlete who, at age 54, will ski in Aspen again this year. Having fully recovered from two knee surgeries, I know what it's like to feel lousy and "over the hill." I had concluded that I was down for the count. Sports would be out, and the ski slopes but a vision from the balcony of the lodge. Fortunately, the feeling was temporary, and the resolve was there. After two years of rehabilitation, and ample nutritional support, and I am back – full of vitality.

I take cold-pressed, organic flaxseed oil. I also take marine-derived glucosamine sulfate and oral systemic enzymes. I add a liberal supply of magnesium, alpha lipoic acid and vitamin E. I greet each new day with vigor. Admittedly, I also take Saw Palmento.

In *The Healing Power of Flax*, you are about to enjoy a trip through key scientific discoveries relating primarily to the healing power of omega-3 fatty acids. You will be compelled by the certainty of their ability to help you feel better, quickly, safely, and completely. There is no doubt about it; essential fatty acids enhance healing, and are the reason why flaxseed oil is listed in my own book The Healing Response as one of the 10 most reliable, proven nutritional supplements to enhance and optimize health—to salubrity, that state of enviable health and well-being.

We know that although we need the omega-6 fatty acids—linoleic acid family (LA)—found in vegetables, oils, seeds, and nuts, our bodies convert linoleic acid into gamma-linolenic acid (GLA), which, in turn, is converted to arachidonic acid (AA). Arachidonic acid is a pro-inflammatory molecule, which means that omega 6 can cause inflammation. The omega 3 family—alpha-linolenic acid (ALA)—found in green, leafy vegetables, flaxseed oil, canola oil, walnuts, and Brazil nuts is converted into eicosapentaenoic acid (EPA), which then is metabolized to docosahexaenoic acid (DHA). Docosahexaenoic acid does not convert to any type of pro-inflammatory mediator. DHA helps boost our immune and hormonal systems. It also helps stabilize our smooth muscles, especially those found in blood vessels that help connect our 250 miles of circulation freeway.

While we need both omega 3 and omega 6 essential fatty acids, we need them in the right quantities and proportions. You will learn why the four-to-one ratio for omega 3 and omega 6 fatty acids is crucial for obtaining optimal, enviable, health. In *The Healing Power of Flax*, you will find simple language that helps you to understand lignans, and how the unique fiber of flax controls hormonal balance.

As a physician, investigative researcher, and educator, I have, until recently, been primarily involved in the study of glucosamine sulfate. I have personally seen outstanding success, particularly in Europe, when this healing nutrient is obtained from a purified marine source. In *The Healing Response*, I emphasize that glucosamine is a building block, a needed repair material for aging and overstressed bodies. Believe me, it is. Take it. But you need more than building blocks to combat inflammation.

Hence, I began my study of oral systemic enzyme therapy, a combination of proteolytic enzymes. Essentially, this type of therapy involves the oral use of bromelain, papain, trypsin, and chymotrypsin. This enzyme combination is an effective, seriously powerful anti-inflammatory work horse, on par with the strongest of the non steroidal anti-inflammatory drugs (NSAIDs), and is safe, with no toxicity. Even the American *Physician Desk Reference* (PDR), under key facts, indicates that these enzymes are said to normalize inflammation and restore tissue to a normal state of function. Not only do they reduce or eliminate inflammation, they can effectively reduce swelling, whereas all NSAIDs are known to potentially cause it.

Effective anti-inflammatory therapies can be found; enzyme therapy is a persuasive representative in this class. Not only do these enzymes ease inflammation, they are biological response modifiers acting through the growth factor system, primarily through thymus growth factor, beta subunit (TGF-beta). Enzymes enhance healing by effectively improving the body's communication system so that what needs to be done gets done quickly, safely, and completely.

Systemic oral enzyme therapy also reduces pain. My patients with rheumatoid arthritis and other inflammatory disorders are always pleased to share their results. My personal quest for information led to the publication of *Healing Sports Injuries Naturally* and *The Aspirin Alternative*. Tools are out there—proven tools to enhance the healing response. We must search them out, pin down the supporting data, and then make those findings known.

It is within this context of the quest for health salubrity that Dr. Joiner-Bey shares his assessment of therapeutic omega-3-containing substances. By bringing adequate, optimal quantities of flax, canola oil, and leafy, green vegetables into our diet, we can balance powerful hormonal systems that act in concert with inflammatory systems and safely prevent inflammatory conditions. Together with other balancing systems, omega-3—particularly flaxseed oil—must be present in sufficient quantities to make endocrine hormones, cell membranes, and other lipid-containing structures, including mitochondria, which is where your energy machinery is located. It is important to note that your brain, which is reading these words, is loaded with omega-3 fatty acids. Without them sustaining the vital process of brain inquiry, your flame would have long died out.

Dr. Joiner-Bey eloquently informs us about important trends in the American diet, most notably a slide into the belief that all oils are the same. While recognizing that oil in our diets is healthy, most Americans believe that both high- and low-saturated oils have their purpose and place in maintaining our health. Our health educators and nutritional engineers have simply downplayed the need to differentiate whether it is omega 3 or omega 6 that matter. This lack of clear direction on fatty acids could be tolerated for a time, but that time has passed. The result is that a marked dietary imbalance has occurred in the unsuspecting American eater. With all the fast food that is deep trans-fat fried, we have quietly been consuming fatty acids that are exorbitantly high in omega-6 acids. In fact, many American diets have unconsciously shifted the ratio of omega 6 to omega 3 to an awkward, unhealthy ratio of 20 to 1, favoring omega-6 oils when a one-to-one ratio would be fine. This pattern of eating has accelerated the production of inflammation-inducing arachidonic acid (AA) to warp speed. It has got to stop. The counterbalance is gone. There is too much tilt and we have a wrecked ship. This is happening as we are seeing more cardiovascular disease, arthritis, a host of chronic inflammatory diseases, and intractable pain syndromes.

I have been seeing patients for more than 25 years; likely more than100,000 patients if I was to count. I have dealt mainly with internal medicine and pain management problems. A lot of these patients had fibromyalgia pain issues. These years have not been in vain. I have been able to educate and help many people to control or solve their health problems. With practice and knowledge, I, too, am getting healthier and better at teaching others to do the same. As I shifted to a greater acceptance of natural therapies, my ability and results have gone way up. Here are some testimonials from my patients about their positive experiences with flax and other natural therapies.

Margorie, a 37-year-old woman with headaches and a pressing job at American Express, says that introducing flaxseed oil into her diet was as an easy as adding an optional ingredient to her lunch-time smoothie. She reports that she does not have as much fatigue anymore—much less than she used to experience during the afternoon. She is also able to exercise when she gets home.

Carol was doing well, but felt constipated and toxic. She did not think clearly as often as she once did. By adding omega -3 flax supplements to her diet, her irritable bowel syndrome improved, especially the bloating, and she felt more naturally herself.

Mark was taking 2500 mg of glucosamine sulfate and 2000 mg of Methylsulfonylmethane (MSM) everyday, yet he still felt stiff. I asked him to cut back on both supplements and use one to two tablespoons of fresh, cold-pressed flax oil every day. He was open to this suggestion. Within three weeks, he felt that he had a 25-percent improvement in stiffness.

These short testimonials are not unusual; they should be expected with flax. What is equally interesting about flax is the rich story of flax lignan—the fiber content of flaxseed. Our bodies need healthy fiber; We don't want the hay and chaff, but we do need the nutrient-rich fiber filled with anti-oxidants. Flax provides this. The history, the research data, and the testimonials amplify evidence that flax fiber helps our gastrointestinal tract, aids in eliminating toxins, and reduces risk of gastrointestinal and many gender-associated cancers. So, we should ask ourselves what health conditions or ills do we have, and what is the potential for flax in our lives?

From my perspective, flax leads to salubrity, the foundation and health principle developed in *The Healing Response*. My patients, at times, tell me I am nutty, fanatical, and even confrontational when I keep telling them that the key to their health is doing things that enhance the healing response. I often ask them, "Why don't you just get better? I want you healed—cured." Sometimes, they get a little irritated, especially when I ceaselessly remind them of the importance of quitting smoking. I also ask them—and you—this fundamental question: "What can I do today to teach you how to enhance your individual, uniquely made, energetically, God-empowered, healing response?

*The Healing Response* lays out 10 principles to get the seeker rolling. The first principle is add flax supplementation to your diet and you empower your energy system . You also get healing energy moving in the right direction, which is the second principle. You have the hormones to drive the metronome, which is number four. You augment cellular communication, which is number six. You provide vital building blocks for multiple repair systems, which is principle eight in *The Healing Response*.

In its first printing in 1999, *The Healing Response* clearly identified 10 reliable supplements, and flaxseed was among them. If you want understandable, convincing arguments to use flax, you will find them in Dr. Joiner-Bey's health-conscious consumer approach. He is an educator at Bastyr, America's premier naturopathic college, and he knows how to teach. This book invites you to take the time to learn, for your own salubrity! When you do, you will be convinced of the role essential fatty acids play in your health, both present and future. You will know that flax is for life!

— *Michael W. Loes, M.D., M.D.(H.)*
*April 5, 2005*

# Part I–
# The Healing Power of FLAX

# CHAPTER ONE

# Flaxseed and Flaxseed Oil— Preventing Cancer, Heart Disease and More!

Why do so many health-conscious consumers nationwide take a tablespoon or two of fresh flaxseed oil every day? Why do others add flaxseeds to their cooking?
Because of the way that it makes them feel!

*There may not be a single nutritional supplement today that can surpass the level of protection against cancer and other diseases as delivered by the combination of flaxseed oil and lignan precursors. It is most unfortunate that so many people are truly missing out by failing to take advantage of this nutrition powerhouse—Mother Earth's richest and most cost-effective source of omega-3 fatty acids.*

Seems as though most everyone has heard the good news about omega-3 fatty acids these days. Hardly a day goes by when omega-3s are not featured on the nightly news, in local newspapers, on radio and television programs, or in health and nutrition magazines. Even many mainstream doctors are expounding on the virtues of omega-3 fatty acids to their patients, family, friends, and the news media. Most recently, the American Heart Association even altered its healthy heart dietary guidelines to recommend that foods rich in omega-3 fatty acids be consumed at least twice a week. And according to the World Health Organization, omega-3 fatty acids are essential to optimal health and life.

## ANCIENT RESOURCE FOR HUMANITY

The flax plant (*Linium usitatissimum*) has been of benefit to humanity for thousands of years. As the source of raw material to make linen, it has been a valued resource for textile manufacturing. In modern times, the seeds of this plant are essential to our health because they provide the richest vegetable source of alpha-linolenic acid (ALA), the plant-based omega-3 fatty acid.

Interest in flaxseed consumption is related to its high content of omega-3 fatty acids but also due to its extremely high lignan content. Although flax is valued for its dietary fiber, protein, mucilage, and other health-promoting compounds, the miracle of flaxseed lies within its omega-3 fatty acid and lignan content. These constituents of flaxseeds, in particular, are potential factors in reducing risk of heart disease, stroke and high blood pressure, as well as diabetes, cancer, autoimmune disease, and almost all types of inflammatory conditions.

The phyto (i.e., plant) nutrients in flaxseed may interfere with the development of breast, prostate, colon and other tumors in humans. The viscous nature of soluble fibers, such as flaxseed mucilage, is believed to slow down digestion and absorption of starch, resulting in lower levels of blood glucose and insulin, and normalizing other endocrine responses. Flaxseed consumption (only 50 grams per day for four weeks) by young healthy adults and by the elderly has been shown to increase the number of bowel movements per week by about 30 percent, thus relieving constipation and possible intestinal toxemia.

---

*Perhaps the most exciting news on flax yet is in regard to breast cancer. A study of 120 women revealed that those with the highest breast tissue levels of omega-3 fatty acids, found most abundantly in flaxseed oil, had the lowest incidence of breast cancer. Further, of those that did develop the disease, they showed the lowest probability of the cancer spreading to other organs, offering hope for women with an existing breast tumor.*

---

Equally important is the role that essential fatty acids found in flaxseed oil play in brain development. Studies on rats and rhesus monkeys reveal that dietary restriction of omega-3 fatty acids during pregnancy and lactation interferes with normal visual function and impairs learning ability in offspring, and may make the brain more susceptible to the damaging effects of environmental toxins and alcohol. When school children in Manitowac, Wisconsin were placed on a diet including flax, their teachers and parents reported improved behavior, higher test scores, and better attendance.

Omega-3 fatty acids have traditionally been supplied in the diet by wild cold water ocean fish, nuts and seeds, green leafy vegetables, sea vegetables, wild game living on green vegetation, and free-range livestock animals grazing on green vegetation. Unfortunately, the advent of industrialized mass production and refining of food has affected the delicate polyunsaturated omega-3 fatty acids such that they are either destroyed, transformed to potentially toxic compounds, or deliberately removed to avoid

### FYI: Most of Us Are Deficient in Omega-3 Fatty Acids

As essential nutrients, omega-3 fatty acids cannot be manufactured within our bodies from other kinds of fatty acids. They must be obtained from the foods we eat. The problem is that we simply do not get enough omega-3s in our standard American diet.

According to Artemis Simopoulos, M.D., author of *The Omega Diet* (HarperCollins, 1999), omega-3 fatty acids are undetectable in blood samples of 20 percent of Americans. As for the rest of us, we are critically deficient in this vital nutrient. Since the body cannot make its own omega-3 fatty acids, the need to include more omega-3 sources in our diet and to supplement our diet with rich sources of omega-3 fatty acids is great.

spoilage and extend shelf life. The role of flax oil and flaxseeds in the diet, therefore, has become even more important in these times of severe omega-3 fatty acid deficiency.

## LIGNANS

Quite apart from flax's omega-3 fatty acids, emerging scientific evidence has begun to focus on another healing element found in the fibrous shell/hull of the flaxseed. Special phytochemical constituents have been isolated in flaxseed that can be converted, after ingestion, to potent cancer-fighting and preventive compounds called mammalian lignans.

> **FYI: Importance of Omega-3 Fatty Acids**
>
> Donald Rudin, M.D., in his book *Omega-3 Oils* (Avery, 1996) likens today's rampant omega-3 fatty acid deficiency to the classic B-vitamin deficiencies pellagra and beriberi of the early 1900s.

Extensive evidence from numerous research institutes has revealed the potent anticancer properties exhibited by these amazing natural plant chemicals. Lignans have been shown to prevent colon and breast cancers by normalizing hormone metabolism responsible for the disease. The American Cancer Society reports that one in eight women will contract breast cancer. Unfortunately, breast cancer may be present for as long as four years before it can be detected by mammography or self-examination. Further, many women are under the misconception that, if they do not have a family history of breast cancer, they need not be concerned. The truth is that the majority of women diagnosed with breast cancer have no apparent family predisposition. These facts call for every woman to implement a proactive approach to prevent the disease. Dr. Ross Pelton, author of *How to Prevent Breast Cancer* (Fireside, 1995), suggests that every woman take at least one tablespoon of highest lignan content flaxseed oil daily to prevent breast cancer.* These recommendations are further confirmed by Samuel S. Epstein, M.D., and David Steinman, M.A., coauthors of *The Breast Cancer Prevention Program* (Macmillan, 1998), who call flax a "profound" inhibitor of breast cancer and other malignancies.

### DID YOU KNOW? There Are Different Kinds of Omega-3 Fatty Acids

Wild fish and flaxseed provide different types of omega-3 fatty acids. Flaxseed provides the omega-3 fatty acid, alpha-linolenic acid (ALA). Some types of cold water fish provide two other kinds, eicosapentaenoic acid (EPA) and docosahexaenoic acid (DHA).

The alpha-linolenic acid in flaxseed is considered to be the seminal or parent compound of all omega-3 fatty acids since it can be converted to eicosapentaenoic and docosahexaenoic acids.

However, sometimes this conversion in the human body is hampered by dietary practices, environmental influences, and even genetics. Both kinds of omega-3 fatty acids are important to human health. One is not superior to the other. They are simply different, and you will want both oceanic and terrestrial sources of omega-3 fatty acids in your daily fare.

---

* Lignan-rich flaxseed oil is unique, as unlike regular flaxseed oil, flax particulate from flaxseeds is retained in the oil, delivering the powerful cancer-fighting mammalian lignan precursors.

## BUILDING A HEALTHY BODY—ONE CELL AT A TIME

It has been a belief among many researchers that disease begins at the level of cellular membranes. Fatty acids are the building blocks for the three major membranes found in cells throughout the body—the outer cell membrane, the nuclear membrane, and the mitochondrial (cellular energy powerhouse) membrane. It is readily apparent from this wide dissemination of fatty acids why omega-3s have such a profound influence on cell function. A healthy diet, rich in omega-3 fatty acids, provides sufficient amounts of omega-3s to permeate the membranes of every single one of the body's one-hundred trillion cells. And the functions of these membrane fatty acids are of immense variety:

- serving as structural components of membranes.
- facilitating inter- and intra-cellular communication.
- regulating insulin production, as well as contributing to the manufacture of other endocrine hormones.
- influencing the response of cells to endocrine hormones, including insulin and the steroidal hormones from the adrenal glands and the gonads.
- providing fatty acid raw materials for the manufacture of local tissue hormones—prostaglandins, thromboxanes and leukotrienes—that influence blood pressure, inflammation, smooth muscle tonicity, and other functions.

Thus, flaxseed oil, with its rich source of omega-3 fatty acids, is an indispensable foundation component of a health-promoting, disease-preventing diet.

### FYI: Flax and Healthy Immune Function

Experimental studies show that adding ground flaxseed and flaxseed meal to your diet, at the expense of dietary corn oil and cornstarch, can boost your immunity to disease.[1] The white blood cells of the immune system become more potent defenders against even tough pathogenic microorganisms.

Dietary lipid (fat) interventions with the right fatty acids (e.g., omega-3s) also have an important role in modulating the onset of autoimmune conditions (in which immune cells attack the body's own healthy tissues, as in rheumatoid arthritis), cardiovascular disease, and cancer.[2]

In fact, it was noted at the 5th International Meeting on Advances in Infantile Nutrition, November 12-14, 1992, Naples, Italy, that many studies have established the adverse effects of saturated fats in humans and in animal models. The increased consumption of many non-flax vegetable oils laden with extremely prevalent omega-6 fatty acids is viewed as pro-inflammatory and suspected as one of the possible causes for the gradual rise in certain malignant tumors, rheumatoid arthritis, and autoimmune diseases. In contrast, omega-3 fatty acids, as found in flax and some types of wild fish, are found to provide protection against cardiovascular disease, rheumatoid arthritis, and cancer. Even the severity of some viral infections may be reduced. Nutritional modification of cellular functions with omega-3 fatty acids offers an attractive avenue to correct, modify, and prevent many maladies.

## FLAX AND YOUR HEALTHY BODY

FLAX HELPS TO:

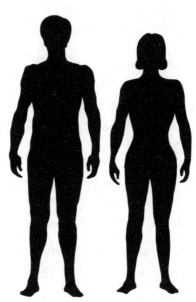

- Support hormone synthesis in the ovaries and testes.
- Regulate pressure within the eyes, joint capsules, and blood vessels.
- Regulate responses of pain, inflammation, and swelling resulting from tissue damage, particularly in the joints and kidneys.
- Mediate the immune response by white blood cells that are produced in the bones and thymus.
- Regulate bodily secretions and their viscosity.
- Dilate or constrict blood vessels leading to and from the heart.
- Regulate collateral circulation leading to the smaller vessels such as those within the brain and leading to the eyes and extremities.
- Maintain proper kidney function and fluid balance.

- Modulate cellular response to endocrine hormones secreted from the adrenal glands.
- Regulate smooth muscle tonicity, such as in the gastrointestinal tract.
- Prevent blood clots by reducing the tendency for the adherence of platelets to each other and blood vessel walls and by reducing the fibrin framework upon which blood clots form.
- Prevent plaque accumulation in coronary arteries.
- Mediate the release of pro-inflammatory substances from immune cells that may trigger allergic conditions.
- Regulate nerve transmission.
- Serve as a primary energy source for the heart.

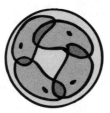

- Influence the rate at which cells divide.
- Maintain the fluidity and rigidity of cell membranes.

- Regulate the transport of substances into and out of cells.
- Influence the transport of oxygen from red blood cells to the tissues.

## WHAT'S AHEAD IN *THE HEALING POWER OF FLAX*

A recent search of peer-reviewed medical journals established a relationship between omega-3 deficiency and more than 40 common diseases.* While I may not cover all of these conditions, I will certainly discuss most and show you how the inclusion of omega-3 fatty acids in your diet can help you to enhance the body's healing response.

1. Acne
2. Agoraphobia
3. Allergies
4. Alzheimer's
5. Angina
6. Arthritis
7. Atherosclerosis
8. Autoimmune diseases
9. Behavioral disorders
10. Breast cysts
11. Breast pain
12. Cancer and its metastasis
13. Chronic viral, bacterial and fungal infections
14. Depression
15. Diabetes
16. Dry skin
17. Eczema
18. Fatigue
19. Heart disease
20. High blood pressure
21. High cholesterol levels
22. Hyperactivity
23. Immune deficiencies
24. Inflammatory bowel disease
25. Inflammatory conditions
26. Kidney disease
27. Learning disabilities
28. Leukemia
29. Lupus
30. Malaria
31. Malnutrition
32. Manic depression
33. Menopausal symptoms
34. Multiple sclerosis
35. Neurological disease
36. Obesity
37. Osteoporosis
38. Postpartum depression
39. Psoriasis
40. Schizophrenia
41. Stroke

### How to Find Omega-3s

Where do omega-3 fatty acids come from? The most fundamental source of omega-3 fatty acids is green vegetation—the phytoplankton in the ocean and green leaves on land. The chloroplasts of plants provide herbivorous animals with omega-3 fats that become concentrated in their cell membranes and fat tissue. Carnivores eating animals nourished on green vegetation also tend to concentrate omega-3 fatty acids in their tissues. For these reasons wild ocean fish, such as wild salmon, mackerel and trout, are excellent sources from the sea. Wild herbivorous game (deer, moose, caribou), as well as livestock allowed to graze in grassy pastures and not fattened on grain (corn), are also good sources from the land. Good land vegetable sources are walnuts and flaxseeds. And the most abundant, economical, and thoroughly researched vegetable oil source is flaxseed oil.

## The Many Health Benefits of Flaxseed Oil and Where to Go to Learn More

**Overall Great Health [Chapter 3]**
Flax is essential to great health. In Japan, researchers believe that the constituents of flaxseed may be the key to long life and prevention of many Western diseases.

**Cardiovascular System [Chapter 4]**
Flax oil fights heart disease by lowering dangerous low-density lipoprotein (LDL, the "bad" cholesterol) and triglycerides, as well as decreasing the tendency of blood to clot inappropriately and preventing atherosclerosis. Flaxseed oil lowers elevated blood pressure in hypertension sufferers. Indeed, only one tablespoon of flaxseed oil daily can reduce both the systolic and diastolic readings in many patients by up to eight or nine millimeters of mercury.

**Cancer [Chapter 5]**
Perhaps the most exciting news on flaxseeds yet is in regard to cancer. Flaxseed products appear to protect against breast, prostate, colon, melanoma, and other cancers.

**Human Behavior and Emotional States [Chapters 6 & 7]**
Flaxseed oil can have very beneficial effects in some cases of depression. It improves the mental clarity of elderly people; provides beneficial effects in the treatment of schizophrenics; plays an important role in helping children with attention deficit/hyperactivity disorder (ADHD); helps to minimize impulsive and violent behavior or emotional hostility in persons so inclined; and helps alleviate postpartum depression, agoraphobia, and bipolar disorder.

**Diabetes [Chapter 8]**
Flaxseed oil helps to prevent the onset of diabetes mellitus, alleviate some of the symptoms of diabetes, and helps to prevent the manifestation of high blood insulin levels that are a hallmark of what is called syndrome X.

**Perimenopause, the Change of Life and Osteoporosis [Chapters 9 & 10]**
Flaxseed oil alleviates many symptoms associated with perimenopause. New evidence indicates flax can be a powerful support nutrient for healthy bones.

**Arthritis, Autoimmune and Other Inflammatory Disorders [Chapter 13]**
Flaxseed oil helps to alleviate allergy symptoms, as well as rheumatoid arthritis, asthma and autoimmune conditions.

**Weight Loss [Chapter 16]**
Flax is a key component in protocols that help many persons lose weight. Flaxseed oil shortens the time necessary for fatigued muscles to recover after exertion.

**Provides Key Nutrient Missing from Vegetarian Diets [Chapter 17]**
Surprisingly, vegetarians may be more likely to miss the vital nutrients in flaxseed than non-vegetarians.

# CHAPTER TWO

# Flaxseed Oil—The Good Fat to Add to Your Diet

America is suffering from fear—some might say unmitigated phobic hatred—of fat. Sure, we know that the wrong fats will cause weight gain, clog arteries, and promote cancer. But we also know that too little fat is also dangerous. After all, what would your poor little sex hormones and cell membranes, not to mention your skin, do without the right kinds of fat? But many people inappropriately hate *all* fat. To gain optimal health, we must be wise enough to realize that there are dietary fats that are essential to life.

## FLAXSEED OIL—FILLING A VITAL NEED

Fresh flaxseed oil is considered to be one of the very best oils for human nutrition. Its value lies in a very rich supply of the two essential fatty acids, alpha-linolenic (ALA/omega-3) and linoleic acid (LA/omega-6), as well as monounsaturated fatty acids (the omega-9 fatty acid, oleic acid, that we usually associate with olive oil). What is unique about flaxseed oil is its high content of the omega-3 ALA relative to omega-6 and omega-9 fatty acids. At 50 to 60 percent, it is by far the world's most abundant vegetable source for the omega-3 fatty acids.

There are many types of distinct fatty acids found in nature (see Figure 1). Linolenic and linoleic acids are considered essential because the body has enzyme systems that can convert these into the other members of their respective families. This means that it would be wise to have both of these fats or other members of both their families to support normal cellular functions. These fats are considered essential for another reason: they must be obtained from food because your body cannot synthesize them. What you eat is what your cells get—no more and no less.

Why are certain fatty acids essential? Essential fatty acids (EFAs) have several vital functions. First, they help to optimize metabolic rate, metabolism, oxygen utilization, and energy production. Second, EFAs and their derivatives are components of membranes that surround each cell, nucleus, and mitochondrion. Lack of EFAs causes cells to have difficulty controlling the substances that enter and leave the intra-cellular environment. Third, EFAs are essential to maintaining healthy cholesterol and triglyceride levels. Fourth, they are indispensable to the normal development of the brain and nervous system in the fetus and young children. In fact, EFAs are important nutrients for the central nervous system throughout our lives and they help to maintain health and well-being (from a psychological perspective) as we age.

Finally, from EFAs, tissues synthesize local hormone-like substances called prostaglandins and leukotrienes. As with the fatty acids from which they are made, prostaglandins and leukotrienes have major regulating functions throughout the body. They regulate arterial muscle tone, sodium excretion through the kidneys, platelet stickiness, inflammatory response, and immune function. Much research is currently being conducted on these compounds because of these important functions, especially inflammatory response.

Unfortunately, it is estimated that more than 60 percent of the North American population is deficient in EFAs, with alpha-linolenic acid far more so than linoleic acid.

I say unfortunate for very good reason: Heart disease and cancer are pathological causes of approximately 73 percent of deaths involving degenerative disease in North America. And both of these diseases are linked to EFA malnutrition. It appears that fat and oil nutrition, which could delay or prevent some forms of heart disease and cancer, has been neglected far too long. This oversight exists no longer. A great deal has been learned about the reasons for widespread essential fatty acid deficiencies and the problems caused by this deficiency. The major obstacle to beneficial change is the massive seed oil industry. In an effort to supply an increasing demand, an elaborate refining process was developed. As you may have already figured out, by the time the oil has been heated, degummed, bleached, deodorized and preserved with synthetic antioxidants, there is very little nutritional value left. Also, the wrong kinds of fats, such as corn and safflower oils, have been popularized—synthetic trans fatty acids found in margarine and those oils which although relatively shelf stable are naturally low in omega-3 fatty acids.

---

**Figure 1:** *Fatty Acids Made Simple*

**The Omega-6 Family**
*Linoleic Acid (LA)*
(Found in vegetable oils, seeds and nuts.)

**The Omega-3 Family**
*Alpha-Linolenic Acid (ALA)*
(Found in green leafy vegetables, flaxseed oil, canola oil, walnuts and Brazil nuts.)

*Your body converts LA into:*
**Gamma-Linolenic Acid (GLA)**
(GLA is also found in borage and primrose oil.)

*Your body converts ALA into:*
**Eicosapentaenoic Acid (EPA)**
(EPA is also found in wild ocean fish oil.)

*Your body converts GLA into:*
**Arachidonic Acid (AA)**
(AA is also found in meat.)

*Your body converts EPA into:*
**Docosahexaenoic Acid (DHA)**
(DHA is also found in wild ocean fish oil.)

## THE SCOURGE OF MODIFIED FATS

The problem does not stop there. The EFAs in oil that have been subjected to the refining process function differently in the body than the EFAs found in fresh, unrefined oils. Refining alters the structure and shape of EFAs. Although they can still fit into the same metabolic pathways, they cannot carry out the same vital biochemical functions. These altered fats can occupy the same positions in cell membranes as normal fats, but the enzymes that attempt to metabolize them will be deactivated. Normal fatty acid metabolism will be obstructed. Not only is it difficult to get adequate amounts of unadulterated EFAs from our modern refined foods, but also any altered and refined oils we eat literally block the absorption and utilization of untampered fats we do ingest. We must eliminate both problems to receive the full benefits EFAs offer.

No other vegetable oil can correct the deficiency as well as fresh flax oil. It contains approximately 70 to 80 percent EFAs with the majority being the hard-to-get and desperately needed alpha-linolenic acid—nature's original omega-3 fatty acid.

## GOOD FAT VS. BAD FAT

So which are the good fats and which are the bad ones? A key to maintaining your body and mind in a state of optimum health is to learn to discern good fats from bad. In Greece and Italy, the typical diet consists of up to 40 percent fat (the same percentage as in the United States). But Greek and Italian men and

### FYI: Flaxseed Is a Food and Cancer Protector

It is best to consider flaxseed oil as a whole food rather than simply a dietary supplement. One to two tablespoons per day is the average adult recommendation. Maximum benefit will be derived if one concurrently decreases the intake of refined fats and other sources of excess omega-6 fatty acids. See our recipe section to learn how to make flaxseed oil a regular part of your diet.

The world's leading authority on flaxseed oil, Dr. Johanna Budwig of Germany, who has been treating degenerative diseases for 30 years, recommends taking flaxseed oil with organic yogurt or cottage cheese (non-fat or low-fat). There are special proteins in these dairy products that enhance the properties of the EFAs. Dr. Budwig has observed amazing success in treating cancer using her oil-protein combination. For additional information on Dr. Budwig and flaxseed oil, I highly recommend her masterpiece, *Flax Oil as a True Aid Against Arthritis, Heart Infarction, Cancer and Other Diseases.*

Just try spreading fresh flax oil on your bread, instead of butter or margarine. It tastes great. The health benefits are profound.

Although many Americans have an unfortunate aversion to seafood, anyone can mix a little flaxseed oil with their yogurt, cottage cheese, or favorite juice. Flaxseed oil could be one of the best whole foods you put into your diet.

women have significantly lower rates of prostate and breast cancer, as well as heart disease. This tells us that it isn't fat *per se* that is the enemy—but the type of fat. The Greek and Italian diet is loaded with omega-3 and monounsaturated olive oil (omega-9) fatty acids. These are the good fats that we don't get enough of anymore because our diet is laden with adulterated omega-6 fatty acids derived from refined vegetable oils, such as corn and safflower, as well as hydrogenated oils (a source of dangerous trans fatty acids) used to manufacture stick and tube margarine and as a baking ingredient.

Good fats can make quite a difference in your lifelong health. In combination with a consistent higher intake of organic vegetables, whole grains, and whole fruits, an adequate intake of beneficial fats found in olive and walnut oil appears to be protective against breast cancer, observes researcher Emanuela Taioli.[3] Not surprisingly, walnut oil is a good source of omega-3 fatty acids, although flaxseed is a far richer source. Similarly, low breast cancer rates in southern Italy are thought to be due to diets that avoid dangerous saturated fats. Interestingly, rates are higher in the north, where French cooking, rich in butterfat, predominates.[4] The diet in southern Italy also lacks the dangerous adulterated, human-made concoction called margarine, a major source of trans fatty acids. Researchers have found a high incidence of breast cancers in rodents fed a diet high in margarine.[5]

## THE ISRAELI EXPERIENCE

Israel has dietary customs that include one of the highest intakes of polyunsaturated and saturated fats in the world. The consumption of omega-6 polyunsaturated fatty acids, found in safflower, corn and other highly processed commercial cooking oils, is about 8 percent higher than in the United States and 10 to 12 percent higher than in most European countries.

In fact, Israeli Jews may be regarded as a population-based dietary experiment exhibiting the effects of a high omega-6 and saturated fat diet. Not surprisingly, there is an extremely high prevalence of cardiovascular diseases, hypertension, non-insulin-dependent diabetes mellitus and obesity among Israeli Jews. There is also increased cancer incidence and mortality, especially in women, compared with Western countries. Studies suggest that high omega-6 fatty acid consumption might be the cause.[6]

Beyond Israel, the problem of consuming high amounts of bad fats at the expense of good fat appears to be of truly worldwide significance. Michael Murray, N.D., comments, "Most people have decreased their consumption of natural, unadulterated essential fatty acids and drastically increased their consumption of refined and adulterated fats and oils."

This trend is most unfortunate. Like Israelis, most of us need to get the undesirable fats out of our diet and incorporate more of the desirable ones.

## ATTACK OF THE KILLER FATS

You've heard about *Attack of the Killer Tomatoes,* that goofy cult film. Well, imagine something far more insidious, killing you slowly without manifesting any clear adverse effects until you are stricken with a heart attack, stroke, or cancer. Dramatic scientific research shows that excess animal saturated fats and trans fatty acids are such insidious creatures, like armed thieves in the night. Trans fatty acids are so dangerous, even the medical establishment is finally beginning to recognize the detrimental effects trans fats have on the enzymes that metabolize fats. Major sources of trans fatty acids are the hydrogenated vegetable oils used in margarine, vegetable shortening, baked goods, and many prepared foods. Another major source is the vegetable oils damaged by their continuous re-use in deep fat frying in restaurants, especially fast food, take-out and drive-through joints. These artificial fats increase risk for heart disease, cancer, diabetes, and other age-related maladies. Removing these obstacles to wellness will go a long way in improving your health.

*Talking about anti-aging, just a tablespoon of flaxseed oil added to your daily diet plus wild ocean fish, such as salmon, eaten twice a week, can significantly extend the healthy years of your life.*

While removing the trans fats from your eating habits, add a tablespoon of flaxseed oil into your diet daily and consume wild ocean fish, such as salmon, twice a week.

## DID YOU KNOW?
### Baked Goods with Flaxseed Taste Great

Muffins, cookies, popovers, buns and bread containing ground flaxseed have been favorably consumer tested at the meetings of the Flax Institute in Fargo, North Dakota, and in the food service system of North Dakota State University, Fargo. In one experiment, banana nut muffins and oatmeal cookies were prepared utilizing either 30, 33 or 50 percent ground flaxseed as a substitute for all-purpose flour. Ninety untrained, randomly-selected college students rated muffins and cookies using a nine-point hedonic (pleasure) scale. Among the researchers' findings:

- Muffins made with ground flaxseed were rated as near optimum in color, flavor, shape, tenderness and texture. The control muffin looked pale in comparison to the muffins prepared with the ground flaxseed.

- Panelists thought that the brown hue of the ground flaxseed gave the banana nut muffins a whole grain look.

- Ground flaxseed cookies were rated near optimum in color, tenderness, and flavor.

- Compared to the ground flaxseed cookies, the control cookies looked pale.

- Both the muffins and oatmeal cookies fortified with ground flaxseed were rated higher and considered more appealing than the control baked goods.

Many bakeries, including one of the largest in the country, have included ground flaxseed in commercially available breads—equating to a recipe for success. Let these test results and commercial trends lay to rest the absurd notion that healthy eating and delicious food are mutually exclusive. What is required is facility in wise culinary skills and creativity.

## WHY YOU NEED AT LEAST A TABLESPOON OF FLAX OIL DAILY

Hippocrates, considered to be the father of medicine in Western civilization, advised people to let food be their medicine. This advice can easily be understood relative to flaxseed oil. Flax is one of nature's most perfect fats to incorporate into your diet because it is rich in two key phytonutrients: omega-3 fatty acids and lignans.

---

*Although many Americans have an unfortunate aversion to seafood, anyone can mix a little flaxseed oil with their organic yogurt, cottage cheese, hot cereal, or favorite juice. Flaxseed oil could be one of the best whole foods you put into your diet.*

---

Accumulating evidence from molecular and cellular biology, animal studies, and preliminary human clinical trials suggests that omega-3 fatty acids and lignans may potentially confer important health benefits related to cardiovascular disease, cancer, and menopausal symptoms. These potential health benefits are con-

---

### DID YOU KNOW?
### What Does the National Cancer Institute Have to Say About Flax?

The National Cancer Institute (NCI) has evaluated milled flaxseed as a component of designer foods.* The results were remarkable. According to the NCI evaluation of flaxseed as a functional food:

- Levels of 1.25 and 2.5 percent flax in the diet stimulated the immune system.
- Flax increased vitamin D levels and increased the retention of calcium, magnesium, and phosphate.
- Ground flaxseed had no negative effects on the liver or intestinal tract and did not lower blood vitamin E levels.
- Flax is high in phytonutrients that have anti-tumor properties and may be linked to a low incidence of breast and colon cancer.
- Flax contains high levels of antioxidants (about 880 parts per million).
- Adding flax to the diet could help diabetic conditions caused by a high-fat diet.
- Based on experimental evidence, it is possible that a 10-percent level of flax in the diet could mimic the results of tamoxifen—the mammary cancer drug—but without side effects.
- Moderately high levels of flax compared to the same level of oat bran were better at lowering triglycerides, total cholesterol and LDL, and had favorable effects on insulin activity.
- Flax is a stable product and stores well.

---

* Designer foods may be defined as those foods composed of one of more ingredients that contribute essential nutrients for health and also protect against specific diseases such as cancer and coronary heart disease.

sistent with epidemiological evidence that incidence of heart disease, various cancers, and menopausal symptoms are much lower among populations that consume plant-based diets rich in lignans and omega-3 fatty acids.[7] People of all ages can benefit from flax. Flaxseed oil has become one of the most successful products in the health food industry due to its preventive and healing properties.

### FYI: Flaxseed Oil Is Easy to Use

Flaxseed oil can easily be incorporated into any diet by using it as an ingredient in salad dressings, as a substitute for butter in oatmeal, as an addition to a blender drink or smoothie, mixed into yogurt, or simply by taking it straight and chased by fresh fruit juice. (See Part III for recipes and cooking ideas.)

The apparent health benefits, including reducing coronary heart disease and preventing cancer, make ground flaxseed a nutritious and healthful addition to foods. Flaxseed flour is a home-grown, renewable, economical, and efficient food-fortifier ideally suited as a designer food ingredient. Food manufacturers are finding flax flour provides value-added appeal to health-conscious consumers demanding more appetizing, attractive products that are also nourishing. Flax is a great tool to boost the nutritional value of many prepared food products.

# Part II–
# FLAX and Your Health

# CHAPTER THREE

# Overfed and Undernourished: Omega-3 Fatty Acid Deficiency— A Major Cause of Disease

Many nutritionists and natural health practitioners would agree that the American population is overfed (in calories, refined carbohydrates, saturated fats, hydrogenated fats, and omega-6 oils) and under-nourished (in pure water, vitamins, minerals, cofactors, and fiber). The eating habits of most people leave them in a state of essential fatty acid deficiency.

Imagine the impact of a shift in dietary patterns so rapid and radical that it adversely affects thousands of bodily metabolic functions simultaneously. Perhaps a worldwide famine, global water or atmospheric pollution and/or radiation could pose such a threat by contaminating or robbing our food of nutrients. The fact of the matter is the scenario given here is not hypothetical, but exists here and now. Though not as obvious as a global catastrophe, the true cause is much more insidious and began with the industrial revolution and the processing of food stuffs to facilitate national and global transportation, packaging and stability.

Throughout human history, men and women have ingested an approximate equal proportion (1/1 ratio) of omega-6 to omega-3 fatty acids. The omegas 6 and 3 are two of forty-nine known essential nutrients. As essential nutrients they cannot be synthesized by the body, but must be ingested directly in foods or in the form of dietary supplements.

The relationship of equivalence between the two omegas is critical because they balance each other to regulate thousands of metabolic functions through biochemical pathways.

Nearly every biologic function is somehow interconnected with the delicate balance between omega-6 and omega-3 fatty acids. As I mentioned, the omega-3s are intimately involved in the control of inflammation, cardiovascular health, myelin sheath development, allergic reactivity, immune response, hormone modulation, IQ, and behavior. A seemingly minor, yet major change in omega balance dictated by dietary ingestion has absolutely deleterious health effects. The rapid change in dietary fat ingestion within only the last 50 to 100 years has bewildered human bio-physiology created to function optimally on equal proportions of polyunsaturated fats.

Diets that provide omega-6 oils at the expense of omega-3s stimulate pro-inflammatory pathways in the body. Omega-3s, on the other hand, stimulate non-inflammatory pathways. As a result, omega-6s have been coined as "bad" and omega-3s as "good." In fact, both are essential for human health and it is the balance of the two in relation to each other that is important. Dominant omega-6s in the body can create a situation that promotes chronic inflammation, propagation of cancer, heart disease, stroke, diabetes, arthritis and auto-immunity disorders.

How did we become so deficient in omega-3 EFAs?

## 1. The Industrial Revolution & Seed Oils

It has long been known that, unless heroic preservation measures are taken, once flaxseed and other seed grains are crushed they soon turn rancid. Because of the high vulnerability of their electrons to oxidation, these precious oils, much like fruits or vegetables, are highly perishable. The husks and germ of grains first began to be removed in the mid-1700s in Great Britain, extending shelf life but removing their vital contents, thereby precipitating overt B-vitamin deficiency diseases, such as pellagra and beriberi. The vital powers of these seed-rich foods were lost. Along came the corn oil craze in the 1950s. The producers of the commodity launched a massive public misinformation campaign, taking out full-page advertisements in the nation's medical journals. This campaign convinced medical doctors that corn oil, so overloaded with omega-6 fatty acids, could prevent heart disease. Most people don't realize that many of the vegetable oils we take for granted today were only introduced into common usage in recent years, since the Industrial Revolution. The development of screw-nut expeller presses allowed the mass extraction of oil from seeds and nuts not commonly used by large populations of people—corn, safflower, sunflower. These are the vegetable oils rich in omega-6 and low in omega-3 fatty acids. As industrialization permeated all aspects of mass food production, the processing of food for maximum shelf life, rather than nutritional value, became the number one goal. A reason to exclude foods rich in omega-3 fatty acids arose. They had to be excluded because they have a shorter shelf life than those with omega-6 fatty acids and hydrogenated fats. Thus, the manufacturers and retailers of processed foods deliberately excluded sources of omega-3 fats in order to maximize marketability.

## 2. Modern Animal Husbandry

The herbivorous animals domesticated as livestock for human consumption were designed by their Creator and Nature to eat green vegetation, the principal food available to them in the wild, not the grain upon which livestock are commonly raised. In fact, virtually all herbivores in the wild live on green leaves, especially the leaves of grass plants or clover, not the seeds of grass plants. The practitioners of modern animal husbandry, in contrast to the way Nature nourishes herbivores, have chosen to rely on grain as a major food source for certain reasons. Livestock grow faster, fatter, and cheaper raised on grain. Unfortunately, their tissue is high in omega-6 fatty acids, in contrast to range-fed animals and wild game, rich in omega-3s. Eggs, once a good source of omega-3s, have also fallen victim to progress. Chickens, like cattle, are fed a diet absent of omega-3s, and as a result their eggs are also deficient. Fish, perhaps the most well-known source of omega-3s, have also been negatively affected. Chances are the fish on your dining table was "farm raised" and did not eat phytoplankton that provides omega-3s.

### 3. Hydrogenation

Refined food manufacturers were quick to learn that omega-3s significantly decreased the shelf life and, therefore, the marketability of their products. Dietary sources of omega-3 were and continue to be purposely avoided in the production of processed foods. Another wrong turn was compounds with the advent of hydrogenation, a process that turns liquid vegetable oils into semi-solid fats. The beauty of the fatty acids in flaxseed is that they won't solidify at room temperature. Thus it remains fluid in cell membranes. When most Americans see the phrase "hydrogenated vegetable oil" on the label of a processed food or vegetable shortening, they really don't understand what that phrase means or its undesirable health implications. Vegetable oils, usually high in polyunsaturated fatty acids, are liquid at room temperature. In order to produce a vegetable shortening which is a semi-solid at room temperature, vegetable oil must be partially hydrogenated. To add hydrogen to the unsaturated bonds of vegetable fatty acids, manufacturers heat the oil in the presence of a catalyst (for example, nickel) and bubble hydrogen gas through the mixture. The result is a man-made "plastic fat" used to give processed foods a particular texture and desired "mouth feel" that American palates have been cultivated to find desirable. Yet, this kind of artificial chemical manipulation of vegetable oils induces undesirable long-term consequences. In their zeal to avoid health problems linked to ingestion of saturated animal fat, people inadvertently ran into other health difficulties. For example, it is intriguing that after the masses abandoned butter and lard for margarine, vegetable shortening, and omega-6 cooking oils, the risk of vascular disease went down while the risk of cancer went up.

### EXPORTING WESTERN ILLNESSES TO ASIA

In a landmark study, Japanese researchers have discovered a leading cause for the advent of Western degenerative diseases in Japan. We now have strong evidence that omega-3 fatty acid deficiency could be one of the most important risk factors for the most deadly, disabling diseases of modern times.

Researchers noticing the proliferation of Western degenerative diseases among Japanese natives asked what had changed in their diet or way of life. Why, they asked, are the people of Japan—who once seemed almost impervious to typical Western maladies and whose life expectancy is markedly greater than that of Americans—suddenly suffering many of the same diseases as other inhabitants of the Western industrialized nations?

The answers have come from Japanese researchers whose recent published work appears to confirm a mountain of emerging scientific discoveries that reveal a major cause for the genesis of degenerative diseases is inadequate ingestion of omega-3 fatty acids. Skyrocketing ingestion of omega-6 fatty acids compounds the problem.

In the West, we may love our sunflower, safflower, peanut, and corn oils, but these are replete in omega-6 fatty acids, and devoid of beneficial omega-3s. These omega-6 vegetable oils are being consumed far more frequently in Japan than ever before, as the American diet begins to permeate the Japanese culture. The results are clear: the Japanese people, more than ever, are becoming susceptible to our Western diseases.

Western degenerative diseases are those characteristic of the degeneration of health and that are linked to long-term consumption of refined and highly processed foods that are a distinctive feature of Western industrialized nations.

These maladies include: heart disease, cancer, stroke, diabetes, arthritis, obesity, and chronic immune deficiency. They have been labeled as diseases of the Western world because Western industrial societies that consume a highly refined diet have a much higher incidence of these diseases, compared to peoples consuming unrefined indigenous diets. Tragically, the American diet is the most refined of all. And to make matters worse, this Standard American Diet (whose acronym ironically is SAD) is being disseminated all over the world with serious pathological consequences.

## OMEGA-3 FATTY ACIDS: 'ESSENTIAL' FOR HEALTH AND LIFE

Why do Western diseases have a striking association with a lack of dietary omega-3 fatty acids? Omega-3 fatty acids are indispensable cellular building blocks. These nutrients must be ingested as food or through nutritional supplementation. There are no enzymes in the human body that can convert other classes of fatty acids (omega-6 or omega-9) into omega-3 fats. If you don't eat omega-3s, you don't get omega-3s. Each of our 100 trillion cells should be supplied with an optimal amount of omega-3 fatty acids. Within the cell wall, omega-3 fatty acids serve to secure structural integrity, as well as facilitate cellular respiration.

In the absence of adequate omega-3 fatty acids, the body must use less desirable fatty acids as surrogates (omega-6 fatty acids and even saturated fats), leading to compromised cellular integrity and overall health.

### FYI: Inflammatory Diseases You Can Prevent or Heal with More Omega-3 Fatty Acids in Your Diet

We now know that an undesirable tendency toward chronic inflammation is at the heart of many of our most common and debilitating chronic diseases. But flaxseed and flax oil can help significantly. Inflammation-related diseases that you can prevent or for which you can induce healing with the omega-3 fatty acids in flax and wild ocean fish include heart disease, rheumatoid arthritis, lupus, and even cancer. There is now some evidence that chronic inflammation predisposes persons to increased risk for Alzheimer's disease. Thus, a diet rich in omega-3 fatty acids may prevent each of these conditions.

In particular, without our omega-3 fatty acids, the body goes into a state of chronic inflammation. The body's inflammatory response is beneficially influenced by omega-3 fatty acids. The inflammatory response was created or evolved as a healing reaction to acute injury or microbial attack. However, if the inflammatory response is needlessly provoked or prolonged, unnecessary damage to tissues and organs of the body will occur. The omission of adequate omega-3 fatty acids in the diets of people among the industrialized nations has created a tendency toward chronic inflammation among many persons. In this case, symptoms of inflammation precede the full expression of diseases such as circulatory problems and cancer. However, as unbridled inflammation tends to perpetuate itself, leading to chronic disease, a vicious circle of inflammation and disease is formed.

The "essentiality" of omega-3 fatty acids cannot be denied. In fact, a deficiency of omega-3 fatty acids in the diet can be considered a reliable indicator or predictor of the risk of disease. Given the research that indicates most individuals are deficient in omega-3 fatty acids, it can be accurately stated that the majority of these individuals will suffer compromised health or premature death as a result.

Making matters worse for the Japanese population is the importation of American dietary habits. This has led to mass consumption of undesirable omega-6 fatty acids, found in high concentrations in common vegetable oils and foods made from such oils. These are the kinds of oils people are eating more and more frequently throughout the nation; thanks to the dissemination of American fast food exports, these unhealthy foods are being inflicted upon the entire human population of the *world*. The massive ingestion of omega-6 fatty acids, out of proportion to omega-3 fatty acids, wreaks havoc on the body's metabolism and inherent protection against deadly diseases.

Put bluntly: The American dietary habits exported abroad are killing the Japanese.

Japanese researchers have documented this dietary shift toward omega-6 fatty acids at the expense of omega-3s. Currently, the Japanese ingest four times as much omega-6 as they do omega-3 fatty acids. This trend is bad enough, but not nearly as troubling as in the United States, where people consume an average of *twenty times* more omega-6 fatty acids than omega-3 fatty acids! Unfortunately, trends in Japan indicate that nation's population may soon match the omega-6 fatty acid intake of Americans.

"Most researchers describe a healthy balance of omega-6 to omega-3 oils as anywhere from 1:1, to 3 or 4:1," notes nutritionist Lalitha Davis, author of *10 Essential Foods* (Hohm Press, 1997). "You probably won't be surprised to learn that the balance of these two essential fatty acids in the body of the average American is about 20:1! This basic nutrient imbalance (way more omega-6s than are healthy in balance with omega-3s) is caused by a diet high in processed and refined foods, grocery store vegetable oils which are highly refined with toxic chemicals, and domestic animal meats."

The commercial extraction of seed oils dominant in omega-6 fatty acids and their widespread use in prepared foods has resulted in an extremely high intake of omega-6 fatty acids in the diet (see Figure 2). Before the Industrial Revolution, people consumed an appropriate one-to-one ratio of omega-6 to omega-3 fatty acids in grains and green foods, and from the tissues of livestock animals and hunted game. The animals consumed then were also rich in omega-3 fats because they were feeding on green

**Figure 2:** *Fueling the Fire*

*Foods and vegetable oils dominant in, or equal in proportion of omega-6 to omega-3 fatty acids.*

|  | Omega-6 | Omega-3 | Ratio |
|---|---|---|---|
| Processed Foods | Varies | None | 100/0 |
| Safflower Oil | 79% | None | 100/0 |
| Sunflower Oil | 69% | None | 100/0 |
| Corn Oil | 60% | None | 100/0 |
| Peanut Oil | 30% | None | 100/0 |
| Walnut Oil | 51% | 5% | 10/1 |
| Soy Oil | 50% | 8% | 6/1 |
| Canola Oil | 24% | 10% | 2.5/1 |

vegetation, the original source of omega-3 fatty acids.

Now, consider the typical fast food meal or prepared convenience foods: French fries, salad dressing, hamburgers and other fried meats are loaded with omega-6 fatty acids and almost devoid of omega-3 fatty acids. And to make matters even more disturbing, the same oil, loaded with trans fatty acids, is used to deep fry potatoes, onion rings, chicken, and other favorites, and it has been re-used day after day for up to three months, when the franchise management finally allows the oil in the deep fat fryer to be changed. The oxidative and other molecular damage done to these already questionable oils is absolutely horrendous—and the same highly reactive molecules in the oil are dumped into our bodies! The oil is laden with rancid, oxidized fats, which generate free radicals, toxic molecules that attack our cellular genetic material and are thought to be the underlying cause of molecular changes leading to the aging process, cancer, heart disease, cataracts, and many other of our most common conditions. And people are daily gobbling food cooked in this waste by the ton. Is there any wonder why we have chronic health problems?

## MONUMENTAL RESEARCH

There has been growing concern by Japanese government and public health officials, as well as a growing legion of health professionals, who have noted a correlation between the adoption of an Americanized diet and a drastic rise in death and disability attributed to degenerative disease. In addition to debilitating illness, the number of allergy patients has increased severalfold in the past 40 years. Today in Japan, one of every three Japanese infants born is diagnosed as allergy-hyper-reactive.

It was this concern that motivated Japanese researchers at Nagoya City University, Faculty of Pharmaceutical Sciences, to investigate the causes of the rise of Western degenerative disease in Japan. The results of their research have been published in the prominent medical journal *Progress in Lipid Research*, occupying 50 pages.[8]

An intensive research study was undertaken which included a thorough review of nearly 500 existing studies related to the issue.

One such review was that of the drastic decline in the health of the people of Okinawa since the advent of American presence on that island.

## THE OKINAWA EXPERIENCE

Citizens of the prefecture of Okinawa used to hold the unique distinction of having the highest longevity among the 47 prefectures of Japan, and, indeed, the world. However, Okinawa was under the jurisdiction of the U.S. following World War II, up until 1972. The Western habitation of the islands began to negatively influence the traditional diet by dramatically increasing consumption of omega-6 dominant vegetable oils. The magnitude of this change was such that by 1975 the amount of vegetable oil purchased per household was twofold higher in Okinawa than in other parts of Japan. The lifestyle of the Okinawan people also shifted from a diet whose major animal protein source was wild ocean fish, rich in omega-3 fatty acids, to meat. The combination of a diet high in vegetable oil and low in fish created a drastic shift in the omega-6 to omega-3 fatty acid ratio. Consequently, there was a corresponding rise in degenerative disease. Sadly, the rest of Japan has reached or surpassed Okinawa in consumption of omega-6 dominant oils, as well as the processed and baked foods that contain them.

By 1990, the longevity of Okinawan males was fifth among Japanese prefectures, which was a drastic decline from the previous top position. The recent trends in lipid nutrition and disease patterns in Okinawa are thus characterized by the most rapid Westernization among the Japanese prefectures. Although the Westernization of cooking and eating habits in Okinawa has preceded the rest of Japan, the other regions have quickly gained ground.

Unfortunately, the Japanese people engaged in these changes failed to realize that they are unwittingly enlisted in a race to an early grave. It is an accurate statement, say these researchers, that the most predictive factor for a shortened life span in Japan, if not the world, is a deficiency of omega-3 fatty acids in the diet, relative to omega-6 fatty acids. The retrospective analysis of the Okinawan diet simply serves as a microcosmic insight into the imbalances in the American diet, which caused Americans to suffer the same fate nearly 60 years earlier.

Perhaps equally as important as the preventive qualities of omega-3 fatty acids are their curative ones. The Japanese researchers found that an omega-3 fatty acid-rich diet, derived from vegetable sources, is helpful in healing breast, colon, rectal and kidney tumors. These findings became even more apparent as the percentage of omega-6s was reduced.

## CHILDHOOD BEHAVIORAL DISORDERS IN JAPAN ARE ON THE RISE

The Japanese have long been lauded for their high intellect and impeccably controlled decorum. However, today in Japan they are faced with escalating incidence of attention deficit disorder and other behavior and learning problems. The traditional Japanese diet, high in omega-3 fatty acids, may have been a contributing factor to the nervous system health and intellectual vitality of these people. It is believed by researchers that 80 percent of the lipids in the cerebral cortex of the brain should be composed of omega-3 fatty acids, with 35 percent in the form of docosahexaenoic acid. For many Japanese children, this severe deficiency has lowered the omega-3 fatty acid concentrations found in brain tissue. These children are more likely to suffer from hyperactivity and similar behavioral disorders.

## FLAX FOR VIBRANT HEALTH AND LONGEVITY

According to Dr. Simopoulos, president of the Center for Genetics, Nutrition and Health, it would take the human body more than one million years to adapt to the radical change in ingestion of omega-6 to omega-3 fatty acids that has occurred only within the last 100 years in America and in the last 50 years for the Japanese.

In other words, this is not a problem that is going to go away on its own. The implications are clear. We must ingest omega-3 fats in our diets and in supplements, while reducing omega-6 fats, to avert otherwise certain degenerative diseases.

Positive changes are occurring in health food stores across America and throughout the world, as consumers are flocking to one of the hottest products on the market—flaxseed oil. A recent nationwide survey in the United States put awareness of omega-3 on par with antioxidants, revealing a 54 percent awareness level among adult consumers.

Likewise, savvy Japanese citizens are utilizing flaxseed oil as a dressing to their traditional morning salad. Incorporating flax oil into a staple, such as the morning salad, is a method that could positively impact lives of countless multitudes of Japanese.

The ingestion of fresh, wild deepwater fish, and toxin-free fish oil supplements also raises the body's omega-3 stores. Consuming the right fish is extremely important. One advantage that the consumption of organic flaxseed and flaxseed oil has relative to some fish and fish oil products is the avoidance of long-term exposure to environmental toxins, such as methyl mercury, common in fish products. This point is critical for women of childbearing age and nursing mothers.

Furthermore, the recent fishing moratorium imposed on China and our own shameful decline of wild Pacific salmon populations underscore the magnitude of fish's decline as an omega-3 fatty acid resource. (There are, however, supplements of omega-3 fatty acids made from marine algae, which could be an important health source.)

## OPTIMAL HEALTH IN THE BALANCE

The ratio of fatty acids in the diet goes a long way in determining risk for many diseases. The difference in proportions between the American and Japanese populations helps to explain why the Japanese, until just recently, have not manifested many of the "degenerative" Western diseases. The ratio of omega-6 to omega-3 fatty acids in the typical U.S. diet is 10:1 to 20:1. But the ratio has been 4:1 in Japan until the recent deluge of American fast junk food. Now the Japanese are eating the kinds of fats Americans do and are suffering the consequences to their health.

The consumption of omega-6s in North America represents 7 percent of caloric intake (about 15 gm daily). The consumption of omega-3s in this population is 0.0 percent to 0.3 percent of calories. Amazingly, people in the upper quintile of that low range for omega-3s (0.66 gm daily) have 40 percent fewer cardiovascular deaths. So even slight improvements can provide significant benefits.

How can we correct this tremendous imbalance? Decrease the intake of omega-6 fatty acid sources. This includes omega-6 vegetable oils, hydrogenated oils, processed foods, products from grain-raised livestock, and farmed fish. Prefer products from range-fed livestock, wild ocean fish, flaxseed, and flaxseed oil. For cooking, use olive oil, which has demonstrated its own health benefits, especially among Italians, who have lower cardiovascular risk despite high olive oil consumption.

I recommend a combination of oceanic and terrestrial sources of omega-3 fatty acids. Flaxseed oil, processed from flaxseed, is a sustainable resource and abundantly available. The only limitation is the proper extraction and handling of the product to protect the delicate oil from degradation.

Perhaps most enlightening are the words of the Japanese researchers excerpted from the study summary:

> In this review, we summarize the evidence, which indicates that increased dietary linoleic acid (omega-6) and relative omega-3 deficiency are major risk factors for Western-type cancers, cardiovascular and cerebrovascular diseases and also for allergic hyper-reactivity. We also raise the possibility that a relative omega-3 deficiency may be affecting the behavioral patterns of a proportion of the young generations in industrialized countries…. It is proposed that dietary intervention with omega-3 fatty acids, and the reduction of omega-6 fatty acids in the diet could successfully reverse the rising trend toward Westernized degenerative diseases in Japan, and the world.

### FYI: How Much Flaxseed Oil to Use Daily

The daily recommenced dose of flax oil is merely one tablespoon (15 milliliters) for every 100 pounds of body weight. In addition, conscious avoidance of excess omega-6 fatty acids in common vegetable oils, grain-fed livestock products, and processed foods is highly advised.

At the same time, beware of oils disguised as "hydrogenated" on food ingredient labels. These oils—also known as trans fats—are linked with increased risk for heart disease. Hydrogenated fats are oils that are heated while being exposed to hydrogen in the presence of a metal catalyst. This process produces an artificial fat that is reasonably solid at room temperature. Margarine is made this way.

# CHAPTER FOUR

# FLAX for a Healthy Heart

Heart disease and its complications are the major causes of death in the United States and have reached epidemic proportions throughout the Western world. Heart attacks, strokes, and other cardiovascular events related to atherosclerosis (hardening of the arteries), blood clotting tendency, and vascular spasm are responsible for roughly 43 percent of all deaths in the United States.

## CAUSES OF HEART AND CIRCULATORY DISEASE

Let's take a look at some causes of this killer:

- Saturated fats in the diet tend to increase serum cholesterol levels, such as low-density lipoproteins (LDLs), the "bad" cholesterol that causes plaque buildup, contributing to atherosclerosis. Thus, saturated fats increase susceptibility to coronary heart disease, angina pectoris, and stroke. Saturated fats also

### FYI: Atherosclerosis Made Simple

Atherosclerosis is a degenerative condition of the arteries. It is characterized by accumulation of lipids (mainly cholesterol, usually complexed to proteins, and cholesterol esters) as well as white blood cells within the artery. There is also the formation of scar tissue that robs the arteries of their elasticity. The atherosclerotic plaque, or atheroma, represents the endpoint of a complex, clandestine, deadly process.

The aorta, coronary arteries, and arteries supplying the brain are most frequently involved in lethal cardiovascular events: heart attacks and stroke.

Heart disease has risen over the past 50 years to become the leading killer of Americans, taking an estimated 750,000 lives per year. Cancer remains the most feared of the so-called degenerative diseases. Yet, the largely preventable malady of heart disease continues to take an even larger toll on people throughout the industrialized world, as more and more countries adopt the unhealthy eating habits of their American counterparts.

inhibit optimal functioning of cell membranes. Trans fatty acids (found in deep-fat fried foods, margarine, and many baked goods) disrupt the functioning of the enzymes that metabolize fatty acids. They also inhibit optimal functioning of cell membranes.

- Local hormone-like substances called prostaglandins are produced from essential omega-3 and omega-6 fatty acids. One of the many important functions of prostaglandins is regulating arterial smooth muscle tone. Any intake deficit of dietary essential fatty acids will disrupt the maintenance of healthy blood pressure, resulting in the production of greater amounts of undesirable spasm-causing prostaglandins and lesser amounts of the desirable relaxing prostaglandins that prevent arterial muscle spasm. A deficiency of these essential fatty acids can lead to elevated blood pressure (hypertension).

- In addition, a deficiency of omega-3 oils, combined with an excess of omega-6s, will cause the overproduction of undesirable compounds (thromboxanes) in platelets (blood components associated with clotting activity) that will cause the platelets to clump together, increasing clotting tendency. Obviously, increased clotting tendency is linked to increased risk of heart attack or stroke. A diet rich in omega-3 relative to omega-6 oils tends to support the production of thromboxanes in platelets that reduce clotting tendency.

All of the abnormalities described above entail either increasing blood clotting tendency or decreasing vessel diameter (via atherosclerosis or vascular muscle constriction). The increased workload on the heart muscle may lead to enlargement of the left ventricle. Is it any wonder why heart disease kills more Americans than the other degenerative diseases combined?

## ROLE OF CHOLESTEROL IN HEART DISEASE

Health-conscious people recognize that high levels of cholesterol in their blood increase their risk of heart disease. Cholesterol is an essential component in the structure of cells and is also the raw material for the synthesis of steroid hormones in the adrenal glands, the ovaries, and the testicles. If your diet contained no cholesterol, your liver would manufacture cholesterol out of triglyceride fatty acids to meet your needs. However, high levels of the kind of cholesterol called low-density lipoproteins (LDLs) can contribute to atherosclerosis.

LDL transports cholesterol from the liver to the peripheral tissues. In the absence of sufficient antioxidants in the diet, LDL can become damaged by free radicals and turn into oxidized LDL. In this modified form, oxidized LDL is an agent that damages the inner lining of arteries, giving rise to atherosclerosis. On the other hand, your body also produces high-density lipoproteins (HDLs) that transport fats from the body tissues to the liver. The HDL cholesterol fraction in your

---

**DID YOU KNOW?**
**EKGs Once Thought to Be Unneeded**

A short 80 years ago, Paul Dudley White brought the invention known as the electrocardiogram (EKG) from Germany to America and was told by his peers that the device held no value given the *extremely low incidence of heart disease in the United States at that time.* Yet only 30 years later, the rise in heart disease in the U.S. was so dramatic that the machine was credited as a most useful diagnostic tool.

bloodstream may be protective against the formation of atheromas in the arteries. HDLs transport cholesterol from the peripheral tissues to the liver for metabolism and excretion from the body.

The LDL-to-HDL ratio (also referred to as the cardiac risk

**FYI: Optimal Cholesterol-Triglyceride Scorecard**

Here are recommended levels of blood cholesterol and triglycerides:

Total cholesterol–less than 200 milligrams per deciliter (mg/dl)

LDL cholesterol–less than 130 mg/dl

HDL cholesterol–greater than 35 mg/dl

LDL to HDL ratio–less than 4.5

Triglycerides–50 to 150 mg/dl

factor ratio) largely indicates whether overall cholesterol is being deposited into tissues or broken down and excreted. The risk for heart disease can be reduced dramatically by lowering LDL cholesterol while simultaneously raising HDL cholesterol levels. Research has shown that for every one percent drop in the LDL cholesterol level, the risk for a heart attack drops by two percent. Conversely, for every one percent increase in HDL levels, the risk for a heart attack drops three to four percent.

One of the first steps in the prevention and treatment of coronary heart disease and strokes is the reduction of blood cholesterol levels. The evidence overwhelmingly demonstrates that elevated cholesterol levels—especially LDLs—are dangerous.

## TRIGLYCERIDES AND HEART DISEASE

Triglycerides, the most common type of fat that people eat, are also now thought to be associated with increased risk for heart disease. In the past, major risk factors identified for heart attack included smoking, high blood cholesterol, high blood pressure and physical inactivity. According to a study published in *Circulation*, however, high blood levels of the fatty triglycerides may need to be added to the list.[9] Elevated triglycerides may be a consequence of other diseases, such as diabetes. Like cholesterol, triglyceride levels can be detected with a blood test.

Researchers say that in middle-aged and older white men, a high level of triglycerides—the chemical form in which most fat exists in food as well as in the body—may mean a higher risk for heart attack. Therefore, the scientists say, high blood levels of triglycerides should be considered an independent risk factor for heart attack. In the study, men with the highest levels of triglycerides were more than twice as likely to have a heart attack when compared to those with the lowest triglyceride levels.

"So far our study appears to provide the strongest evidence that higher triglyceride levels are related to increased risk of ischemic heart disease in men independent of other major risk factors such as total cholesterol and HDL (high-density lipoprotein) cholesterol," says Jørgen Jeppesen, M.D., of the Epidemiological Research Unit, Copenhagen University Hospital, Copenhagen, Denmark.

In an editorial, former American Heart Association President Antonio Gotto, M.D., says that while additional research is necessary to determine whether lowering triglyceride levels can reduce heart attack deaths, the findings make a compelling argument for measuring triglyceride levels as

## DID YOU KNOW?
### What Are Triglycerides?

Triglycerides are the major form in which fat exists in our food—meats, cheese, fish, nuts, vegetable oils, and the greasy layer on the surface of soup stocks or in a pan in which bacon has been fried. The name "triglycerides" arises from the fact that these compounds are made of a three-carbon backbone called "glycerol" with a long-chain fatty acid attached to each of the three glycerol carbons. In a healthy person, triglycerides are normally moved from the intestines to the liver and into storage cells for later use as an energy source.

High levels of triglycerides can influence the size, density distribution and composition of LDL cholesterol—leading to larger, less dense, very low-density lipoprotein (VLDL) particles, which can increase risk for heart attack. An excess amount of triglycerides in blood is called hypertriglyceridemia.

part of an evaluation to determine an individual's risk for heart disease.[10]

"The growing attention to high levels of triglycerides and increased coronary heart disease risk is encouraging to veterans of the 'triglyceride wars,'" says Gotto, dean of the Cornell University Medical School, New York City. "It's also in agreement with another trend in heart attack risk management, namely, the concept of global risk assessment."

Traditionally, people with less than 200 milligrams of triglycerides per deciliter (mg/dl) of blood are considered to have normal triglyceride levels. According to medical texts that guide the interpretation of laboratory results, levels near 200 are those conventionally expected in patients who are middle-aged (40 to 60 years) or older. Between 200 and 400 mg/dl is borderline high; between 400 and 1,000 mg/dl is a high triglyceride level; and greater than 1,000 mg/dl is considered very high triglycerides. Although these levels represent long-held conventional views, naturopathic physicians have concluded, from years of clinical observation, much lower levels are desirable and achievable with natural therapeutic intervention. The latest research is confirming this alternative view.

The normal ranges, based on age group, may require revision. "A very interesting finding in our study was that people with triglyceride levels as low as 142 mg/dl were clearly at a higher risk of heart disease," says Jeppesen of the study published in *Circulation*. "We believe this is of substantial clinical interest since a triglyceride level of below 200 mg/dl is usually considered 'safe.'"

In the study of 2,906 white men who were initially free of any heart disease, researchers found that during an eight-year follow-up period, 229 men had a heart attack. By examining that group of men, the scientists found that heart attack risk increased in those with the highest levels of fasting triglycerides (measurements taken after 12 hours of fasting prior to the test).

"When the triglyceride levels were measured by the amounts of HDL cholesterol in the blood, a clearer picture emerged," says Jeppesen. "Even those who had high HDL levels, which are thought to protect against heart attack, were still found to be at higher risk for heart disease because of their triglyceride levels."

## PRESCRIPTION DRUGS FOR HIGH CHOLESTEROL

While we know that certain drugs do lower cholesterol, the jury is out on whether they actually extend the life span of people with high cholesterol levels. Most studies have shown that people taking cholesterol-lowering drugs are at slightly higher risk of death than people not taking any cholesterol-lowering drugs. That is probably because these drugs tend to interfere with normal functioning of the liver, the organ that is the site of cholesterol manufacture in the body and the target of these pharmaceutical agents. The drug-induced stress on liver tissue is the reason prescribing medical doctors should monitor serum liver enzymes as indicators of liver stress in patients taking these medicines. More recently, encouraging results have been seen from some clinical trials, and doctors are gaining ever-greater faith in these drugs' ability to extend human life span.

In acute, life-threatening situations, pharmaceutical drugs obviously have important uses. Still, in the area of preventive medicine, natural cholesterol-lowering agents are probably a wiser choice. Consider, for example, that an industry-funded study of pravastatin (Pravachol®) reported a rate of breast cancer twelve times higher than among women not using the drug.[11] Bristol-Myers Squibb, the drug's manufacturer, claimed this to be a "statistical fluke."[12] But is it really? As a clinician, such findings do cause me to think twice about recommending such drugs.

A report in the *Journal of the American Medical Association* concluded that commonly used cholesterol-lowering drugs, fibrates and statins, cause breast cancer and other cancers in rodents and that their use "should be avoided."[13]

This finding is of particular importance in view of the growing numbers of patients being placed on this drug, one of four similar ones on the market.[14]

Flaxseed oil is completely nontoxic. The same is not true for medically prescribed cholesterol-lowering drugs. The pharmaceutical industry has developed many powerful drugs to help people lower cholesterol levels. But there are areas of concern when it comes to side effects and complications from their long-term use.

Whereas most pharmaceutical cholesterol drugs are excellent for attacking cholesterol problems, their benefits are limited—and they may also interfere with important metabolic processes. For example, some cholesterol-lowering drugs, known as statins, not only lower serum cholesterol but also levels of the important heart energy nutrient/antioxidant, coenzyme $Q_{10}$. Others have little or no effect on other heart disease risk factors, such as elevated blood pressure or platelet stickiness.

## THE RIGHT OIL FOR YOUR HEART

Researchers at the Harvard School of Public Health say that alpha-linolenic acid intake can reduce the risk of fatal heart attacks.[15] Frank Hu and colleagues studied more than 76,000 participants in the U.S. Nurses Health Study who had filled out diet questionnaires in 1984. Ten years later, 232 of the women had died of a heart attack while 597 had suffered a heart attack and survived.

Women who consumed the most alpha-linolenic acid were about half as likely to die of a heart attack as women who ate the least. They were just as likely to suffer a nonfatal heart attack, though.

Both fish oils and alpha-linolenic acid have anti-arrhythmic effects in animals. So both reduce the risk of sudden cardiac death. But the women who had the lowest risk of a fatal heart attack consumed about 1.4 grams of alpha-linolenic acid a day—the amount you'd get in about half a teaspoon of flaxseed oil.

### The Lyon Heart Study: Diet May Be Enough

Another study, the Lyon Diet Heart Study, determined that increasing the intake of omega-3 from vegetable sources, such as found in flaxseed oil, offers the same degree of protection as increased fish intake.

### Important for People Who've Already Had a Heart Attack

Several studies showing that diet can prevent further heart attacks in patients who have already suffered a first heart attack highlight the importance of omega-3 fatty acids. In the Dietary and Reinfarction Trial (DART) it was only when the intake of omega-3 fatty acids (from wild fish) was increased that future heart attacks were reduced.

In the December 2002 issue of *Lipids*, researchers from the Department of Food Science, RMIT University, Melbourne, Australia, tell us that alpha-linolenic acid from flaxseed "is an important and often underrated [essential fatty acid]."[16] Some so-called experts have "assumed" the main role of alpha-linolenic acid (also known as ALA) is as a precursor to the longer-chain omega-3 fatty acids, eicosapentaenoic and docosahexaenoic acids, found in fish oils. This is not the proper assumption anymore, they add. Alpha-linolenic acid accumulates in specific sites in the body such as fatty tissues and skin, and its conversion to the types of omega-3 fatty acids found in wild fish is absolutely welcomed and important—but by no means its only physiological function. "There is continuing debate regarding whether ALA has actions of its own in relation to the cardiovascular system and neural function. Cardiovascular disease and cancer are two of the major burdens of disease in the 21st century, and emerging evidence suggests that diets containing ALA are associated with reductions in total deaths and sudden cardiac death. There may be aspects of the action and, more importantly, the metabolism of ALA that need to be elucidated, and these will help us understand the biological effects of this compound better. Additionally, we must not forget that ALA is part of the whole diet and should be seen in this context, not in isolation."

This report supports a recent publication from the April 2003 issue of the American Heart Association journal *Circulation*. There, researchers from the Department of Nutrition, Harvard School of Public Health, reported on the association between adipose tissue alpha-linolenic acid and occurrence of nonfatal heart attacks in Costa Rica.[17]

The 482 case patients with a first nonfatal heart attack were matched with an equal number of control subjects. Persons with the highest tissue levels of alpha-linolenic acid had much lower risk of heart attack than those with the lowest amounts. The researchers say, "consumption of vegetable oils rich in alpha-linolenic acid confers important protection against cardiovascular disease."

The diet used in the Lyon Heart Study is often referred to as the Cretan Diet.

The Lyon Heart Study included 605 coronary patients and was conducted to evaluate whether cardiac mortality and morbidity can be reduced by consumption of a Mediterranean-type diet rich in alpha-linolenic acid. This study was undertaken to see if it could reproduce results from the most beneficial diet in another study, the Seven Countries Study.[18] In the Seven Countries Study, such a diet, rich in omega-3 fatty acids, was associated with the lowest coronary mortality rate between the various populations.

But that study was conducted some 30 years ago. In the recent Lyon Heart Study, persons who had already experienced at least one heart attack were advised to consume the following: more bread; more root vegetables and green vegetables (fair sources of omega-3 fatty acids but great sources of vitamins and minerals); more fish; less meat such as beef, lamb and pork; more fruit; and margarine, olive oil and rapeseed oil rather than butter and cream.

The participants were followed an average of 46 months. Individuals in the intervention group consumed less cholesterol; slightly fewer overall fat calories, especially as saturated fat, but more oleic acid and a significant threefold greater amount of α-linolenic acid and other omega-3 fatty acids; as well as more fiber, than did the control population. The intake of vitamin E did not differ between the groups, but vitamin C intake was higher in the intervention than in the control group.

The results were significant. *There was a significant risk reduction of 73 percent in cardiac mortality and morbidity between the intervention and control groups.* If additional cardiovascular events (nonfatal heart

## FYI: How Flax Helps in Heart Disease

Scientific studies have shown normalization of blood lipids (fats) in hyperlipidemic individuals when supplemented with omega-3 fatty acids—as well as decreases in harmful LDL cholesterol, increases in favorable HDL cholesterol, and reduction of triglyceride levels. Blood pressure can also be normalized with the omega-3 fatty acids in flaxseed and fish oils. And we find that arrhythmias (irregular heart beat) and fatal heart attacks are also greatly reduced with adequate omega-3 fatty acid intake.

## Flax and Cholesterol-lowering Agents Work Harmoniously

Are you presently taking cholesterol-lowering drugs? Consuming omega-3 fatty acid-rich foods and supplementing with specific omega-3 fatty acid supplements may be critically important for men and women who are taking one of the known cholesterol-lowering drugs called HMG-CoA reductase inhibitors (also known as statin drugs). These drugs indiscriminately lower blood lipids so drastically that the brain appears to become starved of missing essential fatty acids. Some 15 percent of psychiatric drug reactions could be attributed to this.[19] Further clinical evidence incriminates cholesterol-lowering drug therapy and low cholesterol levels with increased risk for suicide.[20,21] All of this may be attributed to depleted omega-3 fatty acids. It is important to ensure adequate consumption of flaxseed oil in patients on cholesterol-lowering drugs. So even if you are taking cholesterol-lowering drugs, flaxseed oil and milled flaxseed are both absolutely important to put in your diet.

attack, unstable angina, heart failure, stroke and thromboembolism) were combined, the survival rates were significantly improved in the intervention group within the first year.

Even after prolonged follow-up, the protective effect of the diet was maintained. Fewer deaths and other cardiovascular events were reported in the persons whose nutritional patterns most closely resembled the Mediterranean-style diet.

Intake of alpha-linolenic acid "made significant contributions" to reducing this risk, say the researchers. "The results of the Lyon Heart Study suggest that, with a change in diet, it is possible to reduce the incidence of [coronary artery disease]," they add.

### WILD FISH & FLAX: NATURE'S RICHEST SOURCES OF OMEGA-3 FATTY ACIDS

I firmly believe that specific wild cold water fish, such as salmon and mackerel, which are rich in omega-3 fatty acids, should be part of one's heart-healthy diet. So should flax oil. We know they can help reduce your risk of dying from heart disease or stroke.

However, in the October 8, 2001 issue of the *Archives of Internal Medicine,* researchers from the Department of Medicine, Emory University, go even further and favorably compare these foods with cholesterol-lowering drugs.[22]

"Epidemiological and clinical trial evidence suggests that omega-3 polyunsaturated fatty acids (PUFAs) might have a significant role in the prevention of coronary heart disease," they say. Randomized clinical trials with fish oils (eicosapentaenoic acid and docosahexaenoic acid) and alpha-linolenic acid have "demonstrated reductions in risk that compare favorably with those seen in landmark secondary prevention trials with lipid-lowering drugs."

### DIETARY TIPS FROM GREECE AND JAPAN

The two populations with the lowest rates of heart attacks in the world have a relatively high intake of vegetable sources of omega-3 fatty acids: the Japanese who inhabit Kohama Island and the inhabitants of Crete.[23,24]

Typically, Cretans have a threefold higher concentration of omega-3 from vegetable sources, compared to members of other European countries, due to their frequent consumption of walnuts and purslane. Another important dietary factor in both the Kohamans and Cretans is their use of oleic acid (omega-9) containing oils—canola and olive oil, respectively. We now know that LDL-cholesterol, largely composed of oleic acid, is less susceptible to peroxidation. The reason is that oleic acid is monounsaturated, that is, it has only one double bond that can be attacked by oxygen, as opposed to 3, 4, 5, and 6 double bonds found in polyunsaturated fatty acids. The protection of these numerous double bonds with dietary antioxidants is critical. Prompt consumption of these fatty acids after extraction is also important.

Although the oleic content of the diet offers some degree of protection, the rate of heart attacks in the Kohamans and Cretans is much lower than populations that consume *only* oleic acid sources and little vegetable omega-3 fatty acids. The intake of omega-3 from vegetable sources by Kohamans and Cretans is viewed as a more significant protective factor.

## FLAXSEED PREVENTS HEART ATTACK AND STROKE

There are many ways flaxseed (oil and milled) reduces risk for heart attack and stroke:

- Flax lowers low-density lipoproteins (LDLs that, in their oxidized state, cause plaque to build up, damaging the inner lining of arteries) and triglycerides. A recent report from the medical journal *Atherosclerosis* found that flaxseed could reduce cholesterol-related artery disease by 46 percent.[25]
- Flax inhibits excessive platelet aggregation and excessive thromboxane activity, while also lowering fibrinogen levels. Thromboxanes, a family of compounds formed in blood platelets, control the tendency of platelets to stick together and initiate blood clotting. Fibrinogen contributes to the protein infrastructure of blood clots. Persons at risk for coronary heart disease and stroke produce the kind of thromboxane that contributes to platelet clumping and excessive amounts of fibrinogen. Researchers report that alpha-linolenic acid in flaxseed is an effective agent for markedly lowering biosynthesis of unfavorable thromboxanes and fibrinogen.[26]
- The omega-3 fatty acid in flax may prevent fatal heart arrhythmia, according to recent evidence from the journal *Circulation.*[27]

## EXCITING NEW EVIDENCE: FLAXSEED REDUCES C-REACTIVE PROTEIN

I tell my patients inflammation plays an important role in the pathogenesis of coronary artery disease and that they should get their inflammation levels way down—that the way to measure this is with a test that detects levels of the inflammation-marker protein called C-reactive protein (or CRP).

In the April 2003 issue of *Atherosclerosis,* we learn that alpha-linolenic acid is very adept at lowering CRP.[28] Researchers from the Department of Cardiology, General Hospital of Nikea, Piraeus, Greece, recruited 76 men with high cholesterol, following a typical Greek diet. They were randomly assigned either to receive flaxseed or safflower oil. This dietary intervention lasted three months. Dietary supplementation with the flax oil "decreased significantly CRP," as well as serum amyloid A (SAA) and interleukin-6 (IL-6), also inflammation markers and predictors of the ability to survive a heart attack, especially among unstable angina patients. The median decrease of CRP was 38 percent; for SAA, 23.1 percent; and for IL-6, 10.5 percent.

"Dietary supplementation with ALA for 3 months decreases significantly CRP, SAA and IL-6 levels in dyslipidaemic patients," they say. "This anti-inflammatory effect may provide a possible additional mechanism for the beneficial effect of plant n-3 polyunsaturated fatty acids in primary and secondary prevention of coronary artery disease."[29]

> **DID YOU KNOW?**
> **Flax Key to Healthy Benefits of Mediterranean Diet**
>
> An expert workshop convened in The Netherlands recently reviewed the health effects of omega-3 fatty acids and concluded that there is "growing evidence" that consumption of alpha-linolenic acid reduces the risk of heart disease.[30]

## The Missing Key in Healthy Heart Programs

As a naturopathic physician, I believe that quite apart from the usual lifestyle and dietary recommendations you have probably heard about (drinking more pure water, quitting smoking, losing weight, exercising, cutting down on saturated fat) there is one key dietary factor most heart doctors today do not discuss with their patients—and they really should.

If patients would markedly increase their intake of omega-3 fatty acids—if patients would make sure to have an adequate intake of these vital nutrients every day—their risk for sudden death from a heart attack or stroke would be markedly reduced. The scientific evidence is profound.

Let's look more closely at how each of these conditions affects your risk for sudden death and how omega-3 fatty acids may help to markedly reduce this risk.

### Anti-arrhythmic Effects

In a series of studies, intravenous administration of omega-3 fatty acids prevented experimentally induced ventricular arrhythmias.[31] Additional studies show omega-3 fatty acids are able to prevent experimentally induced sudden cardiac death caused by arrhythmias.[32,33] Although the evidence is experimental and preliminary, researchers note, "Increasing evidence suggests that this [same protection conferred by omega-3 fatty acids] may also apply to humans."

In another recent study, the benefits of EPA and DHA vs. alpha-linolenic acid were examined by researchers at the Department of Physiology, Ohio State University, Columbus, for their ability to prevent experimental sudden cardiac death caused by arrhythmias.[34]

With infusion of EPA, five of seven test subjects were protected from fatal heart arrhythmias. With DHA, six of eight were protected, and with alpha-linolenic acid, six of eight were also protected. These

### FDA Allows Nutrient Content Claims for Omega-3 Fatty Acids

The U.S. Food and Drug Administration is allowing producers of food products and dietary supplements containing specific omega-3 fatty acids—DHA, EPA, and ALA—to claim that these products may reduce risk of coronary heart disease. According to an FDA announcement, the "qualified" health claim states that the scientific evidence in favor of omega-3 fatty acids is "suggestive, but not conclusive."

Despite its restrictive language, this FDA announcement constitutes a major breakthrough in this federal agency's awareness about the immense health-maintenance value and disease-preventive benefits of omega-3 fatty acids. This decision is being applauded by consumer health advocacy groups and cancer research institutes that have long recognized the need to restore dietary balance between the over-consumed omega-6 fatty acids and the under-consumed omega-3 fatty acids—an imbalance characteristic of the eating habits of most Americans. These new labeling guidelines will allow consumers to learn which foods are rich in specific types of omega-3 fatty acids.

The enactment of these new decisions is a positive outgrowth of the FDA's streamlined notification procedure to provide consumers with timely health information for better nutritional choices.

results indicate that when it comes to prevention of heart arrhythmias, both fish oils and flax are equivalent. Indeed, based on the experimental evidence, the researchers conclude, "purified omega-3 fatty acids can prevent ischemia-induced ventricular fibrillation."

The ability of both EPA and alpha-linolenic acid to protect against heart arrhythmia was further confirmed in yet another recent experimental study published in *The European Journal of Pharmacology.*[35]

## Decreasing Platelet Aggregation

Like aspirin, omega-3 fatty acids inhibit platelet aggregation, helping to prevent undesirable blood clotting—although benefits will be even more dramatic if rich sources of omega-3 fatty acids such as salmon and flax oil are substituted for fatty foods like fatty cuts of meat and whole-fat dairy desserts.[36]

## Normalizing Blood Pressure

The simple process of having blood flow through the arteries causes wear and tear. Even young persons in their twenties show signs of this wear and tear, as we learned in autopsy reports of young veterans of the Korean War whose arteries suffered their most extensive damage above the branches in arteries, where blood flow is most turbulent.[37] However, high blood pressure, which causes the vessels to work much harder and more forcefully, imposes extensive stress on arterial walls and potential damage. If your diastolic blood pressure is above 105, your risk is doubled for heart attack, quadrupled for stroke.

In a 1986 report from the *American Journal of Clinical Nutrition,* among 399 men with an average age of 47, it was found that for every one percent increase in the body's content of alpha-linolenic acid, they experienced a corresponding decrease of 5 mmHg (millimeters of mercury) in the systolic, diastolic, and composite mean arterial blood pressure.[38] (The richest source of alpha-linolenic acid, which is considered the parent compound of all of the omega-3 fatty acids, is flaxseed.)

Cardiovascular tissue knows exactly how to use omega-3s to optimize health. One type of eicosanoid, thromboxane $A_3$, which is produced in platelets, helps to relax the arteries and help them to expand, allowing more blood flow. However, the fats typically consumed in the standard American diet, including saturated fats and all-too-plentiful omega-6 fatty acids (found in processed vegetable oils), induce production of thromboxane $A_2$ which causes arterial constriction.

## Lowering Inflammation

One way aspirin exerts its beneficial effects on heart health is by lowering overall inflammatory states throughout the body. Unfortunately, although chronic inflammation is a major heart attack risk factor, the public barely knows about this important contributor to sudden death, including second heart attacks. It has been shown that overall bodily inflammation, as measured by serum C-reactive protein, increases risk of a heart attack by threefold and risk of stroke by twofold.[39] Fortunately, omega-3 fatty acids reduce overall bodily inflammation—without the harsh effects that aspirin has on the stomach lining.[40]

### Free Radical Damage

The buildup of plaque on the inner lining of arteries increases risk for sudden blood clots. Free radicals have been implicated in the generation of arterial plaque. Free radicals damage LDL cholesterol in a process called oxidation. According to the "free radical" theory of atherosclerosis, free radicals in the blood, including oxidized LDL, damage the inner lining (intima) of the arteries at the major blood flow stress points. Damage to the intima exposes the underlying connective tissue to the blood. Platelets immediately recognize that a "wound" in the arterial tissue has occurred and attach themselves to the damaged area in an effort to heal the tissue. Cholesterol, minerals, proteins and other blood constituents adhere to the platelet foundation, forming the atheroma plaque. The type of plaque most likely to rupture and cause a clot covers large areas, and may be chronically inflamed. We call this "vulnerable plaque." In a heart attack, deposits of plaque may dislodge, causing debris to be dumped into the bloodstream. This triggers blood clot formation and a subsequent heart attack or stroke.

## WISDOM FROM THE TUNDRA

There is ample evidence that omega-3 fatty acids inhibit plaque buildup, as well as subsequent clots. Our first insight into the beneficial effects of omega-3 fatty acids comes from the work of Danish scientists H.O. Bang and Jorn Dyerberg who discovered that Eskimos consuming their traditional diet, which is rich in cold water fish and marine mammals, have very low rates of heart attacks. Having reviewed a decade's worth of medical records at a Greenland hospital, among some 2,000 persons there was not a single death caused by heart attack. In publishing their findings, the researchers noted, "We believe that [eating more omega-3 fatty acids] could be as effective in the prevention of cardiovascular disease as the large-scale use of drugs."[41]

Omega-3 fatty acids have other important benefits. It is known that high levels of substances called platelet-activating factor, interleukin-1, tumor necrosis factor and leukotriene $B_4$ mediate inflammation. Omega-3 fatty acids reduce the production of each of these chemicals, thus markedly reducing inflammatory processes. In particular, the lignans in flax possess anti-platelet activating factor (PAF) activity and exert antioxidant effects, offering protection against oxidative damage and preventing plaque buildup.

In an experimental study from the Department of Physiology, College of Medicine, University of Saskatchewan, Saskatoon, Canada, the effects of dietary flaxseed on a high-cholesterol diet were investigated.[42] Rabbits fed a high-cholesterol diet without flax displayed increased serum levels of total cholesterol, which was associated with a marked development of atherosclerosis. The addition of flaxseed reduced the development of atherosclerosis by 46 percent. "Dietary flaxseed supplementation could, therefore, prevent hypercholesterolemia-related heart attack and strokes," according to the report.

There are other ways omega-3 fatty acids prevent clots. The formation of a clot requires the clumping of platelets and a fibrous network made from the blood protein fibrinogen. It is known that people with high fibrinogen levels experience some five times greater risk for heart attack and premature death. Omega-3 fatty acids make platelets less sticky and decrease fibrinogen production.[43]

## ALPHA-LINOLENIC ACID PREVENTS SECOND HEART ATTACK AND STROKE

Have you had a heart attack already? Then, when you do consume fat (which we all must do to some extent), flax's alpha-linolenic acid could be one of your heart's very best friends. In a heart attack prevention trial, European doctors compared the effect of a Mediterranean alpha-linolenic acid-rich diet to the usual post-heart attack diet, as recommended by the American Heart Association.[44]

After a first heart attack, 302 patients were randomly assigned to the experimental Mediterranean diet, and 303 to the usual post-heart attack diet. Patients were seen eight weeks after being assigned to their diet group and each year for five years. The Mediterranean group consumed significantly less saturated fat, cholesterol, and linoleic acid but more oleic (from olive oil) and alpha-linolenic acids (which was confirmed by measurements in plasma). In the Mediterranean diet group, plasma levels of vitamin E and vitamin C were also increased. Serum lipids, blood pressure, and body mass index remained similar in the two groups.

After a mean follow-up of 27 months, there were 16 cardiac deaths in the regular diet group and only 3 in the Mediterranean group; there were 17 nonfatal second heart attacks in the regular diet group and only 5 in the Mediterranean diet group. Overall, 20 deaths occurred in the regular diet group and only 8 in the Mediterranean group. The researchers concluded that, "an alpha-linolenic acid-rich Mediterranean diet seems to be more efficient than presently used diets in the secondary prevention of coronary events and death."

Flax's alpha-linolenic acid may also be key to stroke prevention. In an experimental study, the life span of rodents that suffered from high blood pressure and propensity for strokes was increased by

### DID YOU KNOW?
### Sudden Death from Heart Attack in Women

People tend to think of cardiovascular disease as a male affliction because the symptoms show up ten years earlier in men. But women catch up after menopause. For women, heart disease may not be an issue prior to menopause, thanks to the artery-sparing effects of female hormones.

But following menopause, women's risk for heart disease increases dramatically and becomes similar to that of men. In fact, statistically, more women die from heart attacks than men. And five times more women die from a heart attack than from breast cancer. Fortunately, alpha-linolenic acid found in flax may be one of women's best friends when it comes to heart protection.

In the May 1999 *American Journal of Clinical Nutrition,* researchers from the Department of Nutrition, Harvard School of Public Health, reported results from a 10-year study that obtained heart disease data from a pool of 76,283 women.[45] After adjustment for age, standard heart disease risk factors and dietary habits, "a higher intake of alpha-linolenic acid was associated with a lower relative risk of fatal [heart disease]," say these scientists. In fact, women with the highest intake of alpha-linolenic acid reduced their heart disease mortality rate by a significant 55 percent. Interestingly, the researchers found that these women were obtaining their alpha-linolenic acid from mayonnaise and salad dressings—but pure flax oil would be a better choice. Some salad dressings may also contain some of the harmful fats.

17 percent when given a seed oil rich in alpha-linolenic acid.[46] Their systolic blood pressure was lowered by 10 percent. The rodents' blood platelets were also less sticky and less prone to form a stroke-causing clot.

### STROKE: A PREVENTABLE MEDICAL MALADY WITH OMEGA-3 FATTY ACIDS

Cerebral vascular stroke is the most common cause of neurological damage in the industrialized Western world, and is a leading cause of death and disability in these countries. Formerly proud, productive and independent persons can be reduced to becoming totally or partially dependent on others for the most basic of needs. The financial, as well as emotional, impact on the family members of these victims is staggering. The most common cause of cerebral vascular stroke is the formation of a clot occluding blood flow to brain tissue. Prolonged cessation of blood flow to the brain causes oxygen depravation and death of brain tissue in the affected area. Another cause of stroke is the rupturing of a blood vessel in the brain. The location and severity of the stroke determines the level of infirmity, resulting in partial paralysis, inability to speak, and in severe cases, brain death.

A practical approach to preventing cerebral vascular stroke would ultimately save millions of dollars in health care costs, while significantly reducing the pain and suffering on behalf of the patients and family members. The Food and Drug Administration (FDA) has just approved a new drug for the treatment of stroke. Unfortunately, you have to have a stroke first, before being administered the medicine. If the drug is not given within a very narrow window of time, it can actually worsen the stroke. Modern medicine has provided very little in the way of preventing this disabling and sometimes fatal affliction. The message here is that we must assume responsibility for our health by initiating dietary, supplemental, and lifestyle changes to prevent stroke and other medical infirmities.

A sensible solution in the prevention of stroke is found in both the strengthening of blood vessels and lowering the abnormal clotting tendency of the blood. This two-pronged approach helps to prevent the rupture of cerebral blood vessels, while at the same time preventing blood platelets from clumping together in the formation of a clot.

Flavonoid compounds found in select fruits and vegetables have been found to improve the integrity of blood vessels, as has vitamin C. Of particular value are the purple-blue and dark red flavonoids of the anthocyanidin family found in grape seed extract (Vitis vinifera) and bilberry (Vaccinium myrtillus). Antioxidant nutrients further protect blood vessels from damage by free radicals.

Research on omega-3 fatty acids found most abundantly in flaxseed oil might offer the most hope yet. Study results reported in the May 1995 issue of the American Heart Association's Stroke suggest the omega-3 alpha-linolenic acid may protect against stroke. Analyzing data from the long-running Multiple Risk Factor Intervention Trial, researchers found that participants with high blood levels of alpha-linolenic acid had a 37 percent lower risk of stroke, presumably because of the fatty acids' ability to reduce the platelet "stickiness" and blood clotting. Omega-3 fatty acids essentially prevent blood platelets from clumping together and forming a dangerous clot by making them "slippery."

## FLAX VS. FISH OILS: MUST WE CHOOSE ONE OVER THE OTHER?

Although a great deal of advertising money and marketing effort is spent on attempting to convince consumers that fish oils are superior to flax as a source of omega-3 fatty acids, the fact is heart-smart consumers should take advantage of the unique characteristics of both fish and flax. Each makes a unique and valid contribution to circulatory and heart health.

### Differences Between Flax and Fish Oil

Fish oils provide two omega-3 fatty acids called eicosapentaenoic acid (EPA) and docosahexaenoic acid (DHA). Flax provides alpha-linolenic acid (ALA). Scientists consider alpha-linolenic acid to be the parent compound or precursor of both EPA and DHA. The body can convert alpha-linolenic acid into both EPA and DHA. One often cited drawback to flax oil, however, is that the efficiency of this conversion can be reduced due to factors that interfere with the activity of enzymes involved in the conversion. Among the areas of concern that can inhibit conversion of alpha-linolenic acid to EPA and DHA:

- high intake of omega-6 fatty acids (which are found in commonly used vegetable oils and processed foods);
- significant alcohol intake;
- deficiency of enzyme cofactors, such as vitamins $B_3$, $B_6$, and C; zinc; and magnesium;
- trans fatty acids in the diet;
- naturally slow or diminished enzyme activity.

On the other hand, of course, low-quality fish oils can contain contaminants and free radical-generating peroxides.

### Lower Blood Pressure with Flax

High blood pressure or hypertension refers to a reading of greater than 140/90 millimeters of mercury (mmHg). An elevated blood pressure is one of the major risk factors for a heart attack or stroke. Since heart disease and strokes account for over 43 percent of all deaths in the U.S., it is very important to keep blood pressure in the normal range. Over 60 million Americans have high blood pressure. Dietary factors appear to be the primary reason.

Most health experts stress safe, natural pathways for lowering blood pressure whenever possible to avoid the complications of pharmaceutical drugs.

More than 60 double-blind studies have confirmed that supplements rich in omega-3 fatty acids (of which flaxseed's alpha-linolenic acid or ALA is one of the key members) are beneficial for lowering blood pressure.[47,48,49] We also know taking the equivalent of one tablespoon of flaxseed oil daily can lower both systolic and diastolic blood pressure readings by up to 9 mmHg.[50] In fact, for every one percent increase in the concentration of ALA in the body, persons can expect to see a decrease of 5 mmHg in both their systolic and diastolic blood pressure.[51]

| Best Sources of Omega-3 Fatty Acids in Wild Fish | |
| --- | --- |
| Fish | Amount per 100 grams of raw fillet |
| Rainbow trout | 1.1 |
| Cisco | 1.1 |
| Pacific mackerel | 1.1 |
| Atlantic herring | 1.1 |
| Pacific herring | 1.2 |
| Sardine | 1.2 |
| American eel | 1.2 |
| Atlantic halibut | 1.3 |
| Sablefish | 1.3 |
| Atlantic salmon | 1.4 |
| Lake trout | 1.4 |
| Anchovy | 1.4 |
| Coho salmon | 1.5 |
| Pink salmon | 1.5 |
| Atlantic mackerel | 1.9 |
| King salmon | 1.9 |
| Dogfish | 1.9 |
| Sockeye salmon | 2.7 |

Source: Nettleton, Joyce A. *Seafood Nutrition— Facts, Issues and Marketing of Nutrition in Fish and Shellfish.* Huntington, NY: Osprey Books, 1985.

However, often lost in the discussion is the fact that alpha-linolenic acid has its own heart-health properties that make the addition of flax to the diet particularly beneficial. Substantial clinical validation tells us a combination of both land and sea sources of omega-3 fatty acids is the best way to go.

Certainly, most persons would be better off dining on a broiled, wild fish from an omega-3 fatty acid-rich source, such as wild salmon, when dining out. But, the reality is that many Americans simply don't *like* eating fish. Thus, researchers writing in 1996 conclude that, "Most American consumers, however, given their preference for meat, will not realize the benefits of a fish-rich diet."[52]

However, in their study, these researchers found that substituting measured amounts of flaxseed oil for measured amounts of olive and corn oils could produce virtually an equivalent effect to that of fish in terms of favorably down-modulating synthesis of blood flow-impairing eicosanoids, such as thromboxane $A_3$ and prostacyclin: "This study demonstrates that dietary alpha-linolenic acid is an effective modulator of thromboxane and prostacyclin biosynthesis. Therefore, we can expect that the eicosanoid-mediated effects of alpha-linolenic acid are similar to those elicited by marine lipids."

Dr. Michael Murray, author of *Encyclopedia of Nutritional Supplements* (Prima, 1996), concludes, "Alpha-linolenic acid produces many of the same effects as EPA and several of its own. . . . Flaxseed oil provides a significant cost saving as well. The dosages effective in lowering cholesterol levels when using fish oil supplements range from 5 to 15 grams per day. Since most commercial products contain 500 milligrams of fish oil per capsule, this means a daily dose of 10 to 30 capsules at an average monthly cost of $40 to $100. At a similar dosage, flaxseed oil costs between $6 and $18 per month."

One great way to go, especially if you suffer from high blood pressure, is to take six flaxseed oil capsules three times daily, and to be sure to substitute wild salmon for dinner or lunch three to four times a week. I also recommend flax-based cereals with soy milk as another savvy heart-health dietary change.

Other persons may prefer to take both flaxseed and high-quality laboratory-tested fish oil capsules.

Flaxseed oil can be used for many types of dressings and other easily prepared foods, including delicious fruit smoothies (see Part III). However, I strongly recommend that unless you are consuming flaxseed daily in your recipes, you supplement your diet with flaxseed oil or capsules. Take two tablespoons of oil daily, or six capsules, three times daily.

# CHAPTER FIVE

# Reduce Cancer Risk
# with Flaxseed

Could a flaxseed muffin or two a day keep breast and prostate cancer at bay? The news on flax and cancer prevention is very positive. If you consumed flax oil or flaxseed for no other reason than cancer prevention, you would be doing a wonderful thing for your health.

In particular, flaxseed holds a special role for the prevention of pancreatic, colon, breast and prostate cancers, as well as prevention of the spread of melanoma.

The Mediterranean diet, traditionally consumed in Greece and regions of Italy, emphasizes whole grains, fruits, vegetables, wild fish, and olive oil with limited meat and dairy (in the form of cheese). It is not a particularly low-fat diet. In fact, the average daily intake of fat for Greek women is 40 percent of total calories, a figure roughly equivalent to the American.[53] Yet, Greek women have much lower breast cancer rates than their American counterparts. Together with a higher intake of vegetables, whole grains, and fruits, a high intake of neutral or beneficial fats found in olive and walnut oils appears to be protective.[54]

Similarly, low breast cancer rates in southern Italy are thought to be due to diets that avoid dangerous saturated fats, whereas rates are higher in the north where French cooking, rich in butterfat, predominates.[55] The absence of margarine, a major source for dangerous trans fatty acids, from the southern diet is also important, as researchers have found a high incidence of breast cancers in rodents fed a diet high in margarine.[56]

Moving to another country, Israel has one of the highest intakes of polyunsaturated and saturated fats in the world. The consumption of omega-6 polyunsaturated fatty acids, which are found in safflower, corn and other highly processed commercial cooking oils, is about 8 percent higher in Israel than in the United States and 10 to 12 percent higher than in most European countries.

Not surprisingly, there is an extremely high prevalence of cardiovascular diseases, hypertension, non-insulin-dependent diabetes mellitus and obesity among Israeli Jews. There is also an increased cancer incidence and mortality rate, especially for women, compared with Western countries. Studies suggest that high omega-6 fatty acid consumption might be the cause.[57]

We must take these findings very seriously if we are to enjoy optimal health. For American women and men, emphasizing the good fats, such as those from wild fish and unrefined flaxseed and walnut oils, is critical for maintaining normal cell growth and reproduction. Each of these sources is rich in omega-3 fatty acids, which have shown suggestive evidence that they can reduce risk for several types of cancers.

## FLAX AND BREAST CANCER

A muffin a day—with 50 grams of ground flaxseed—could keep breast cancer at bay, according to a new Canadian study. The researchers found there was a "slowing down in tumor growth" in breast cancer patients fed flaxseed muffins.[58]

"Our results are very exciting because this is the first time anyone has demonstrated these changes in breast cancer with any dietary component," said Dr. Paul Goss, director of the Breast Cancer Prevention Program at Princess Margaret Hospital and the Toronto Hospital.

Earlier animal studies have shown that flaxseed has anticancer properties, but the researchers were surprised by how potent the effect appears to be in people.

"It encourages us to believe this is a very significant biological effect in women and we are heading towards more definitive proof that dietary flaxseed may prevent breast cancer," Goss said.

Goss presented his research team's finding at an international breast cancer conference in San Antonio, Texas. The study involved 50 women who had been recently diagnosed with breast cancer. While waiting for their surgery, the women were divided into two groups. One group received a daily muffin containing 50 grams of ground flaxseed (equivalent to about 30 milliliters of flax oil or two tablespoons of milled flaxseed a day). The others were prescribed ordinary muffins.

### An Amazing Study

Every woman concerned with breast cancer needs to be aware of an amazing landmark study conducted by Jeffrey Bland, Ph.D., and Ewan Cameron, M.D., more than a decade ago. Using a special strain of laboratory mouse known for its genetic predisposition for breast cancer, Drs. Bland and Cameron took 300 of these mice and divided them into six experimental groups of 50 mice each. The control group received only the lard-based chow as the exclusive dietary source. The remaining five groups were all treated with a known carcinogenic agent. In addition, each of these groups received a different dietary source of fatty acids. One group received omega-3s from flax and another received omega-3s from fish. The remaining groups received fatty acids from a variety of vegetable oils commonly consumed by humans in the United States. Neither Bland nor Cameron knew which group received which intervention; only the laboratory technicians knew. Weeks later, the researchers were informed that of the six groups, two exhibited 100 percent survival and the remaining four groups had 100 percent mortality. Bland and Cameron guessed that one of the survival groups was the control group. They were wrong. To their surprise, all the control animals, fed only lard-based laboratory mouse chow, died of the genetically induced breast cancer. The two groups that displayed 100 percent survival, despite genetic cancer risk and carcinogen exposure, were the flax and fish omega-3 groups. All other groups fed typical vegetable oil fatty acids had 100 percent mortality. These results were so incredible, the editors of medical journals in which the researchers wanted to publish an article on this experiment absolutely insisted that the experiment be repeated. It was, and with the same results. Clearly, this is a strong indication that when we improve the quality of the fatty acids on cell, nuclear, and mitochondrial membranes using omega-3s, we have a powerful beneficial influence on how our cells respond to pathological genetic tendencies and environmental influences.

When their tumors were removed—usually within 40 days of diagnosis—the researchers examined them for signs of how fast the cancer cells had been growing. It turned out that the women who had received the flaxseed muffins had much slower-growing tumors than the others. No doubt, these women were much more likely to survive their cancers.

The American Cancer Society reports that one in eight women will contract breast cancer. Unfortunately, breast cancer may be present for as long as four years before it can be detected by mammography or self-examination. Further, many women are under the misconception that if they do not have a family history of breast cancer, they need not be concerned. The truth is the majority of women today who are diagnosed with breast cancer show no family predisposition. Why are so many women without medically significant family history succumbing to this disease? In the view of alternative practitioners, a combination of circumstances, unknown to previous generations, makes modern women more susceptible to this disorder. The abundance of chemicals in the environment that have estrogenic effects, nutritional deficiencies in essential fatty acids, vitamins, and minerals, and excessive intake of omega-6 fats, trans fatty acids, and refined carbohydrates—all of these factors combine to increase susceptibility to breast cancer in American women. The above facts call for every woman to implement a proactive approach to prevent the disease.

We suggest that every woman take at least one tablespoon of highest lignan content flaxseed oil daily to reduce her risk of breast cancer. In addition, the wise woman would also add ground flaxseeds to her diet, as an addition to hot breakfast cereal, home baked goods, soups, and other dishes, to receive the protective benefit of additional lignans in her diet. The addition of a flaxseed lignan concentrate is also highly recommended.

Highest lignan content flaxseed oil is unique. Unlike regular flaxseed oil, with highest lignan content products, flax particulate from flaxseeds is retained in the oil.

## FLAXSEED: NATURE'S RICHEST SOURCE OF PLANT LIGNANS

Beginning in the 1980s, consumers were advised by the Surgeon General of the United States and the National Academy of Sciences that diets low in saturated fat and high in fiber could be beneficial to their health. This advice was driven by new health statistics. For example, five of the ten leading causes of death in the United States—including coronary heart disease, some types of cancer, stroke, diabetes and atherosclerosis—were related to dietary imbalances.

Consequently, the Surgeon General advised consumers to lower their saturated fat and cholesterol intake, and, at the same time, increase their consumption of whole grains, vegetables and fruits. This new information convinced the National Cancer Institute (NCI) to undertake a $20.5 million program to learn more about natural plant chemicals (phytochemicals) in certain food groups that may prevent cancer.

One of the first and most promising foods to be studied was flaxseed. It had been previously discovered that flaxseed contained phytochemicals known as lignans within the cell matrix of its seed. Much of the interest surrounding plant lignans is based on the suspected association between them and the low incidence of breast and colon cancers of those consuming a plant- and grain-based vegetarian diet. Lignans are converted, by bacteria in the colon, into the compounds enterolactone and enterodiol that have protective effects against breast cancer and other malignancies. Flaxseed, in particular, contains 100 to 800 times more plant lignans than its closest competitors, wheat bran, rye, buckwheat, millet, soybeans, and oats.

The lignans found in flaxseed, once consumed and converted to the mammalian lignans enterolactone and enterodiol, are then absorbed through the intestinal mucous membrane into the bloodstream. The mammalian lignans bind with estrogen receptors on cells throughout the body, reducing the effect of women's estrogen hormones by blocking the receptors the hormones activate. In addition, these compounds are believed to induce an increased production of sex hormone binding globulin, which controls the overall availability and influence of women's estrogens. Sex hormone binding globulin (SHBG) regulates estrogen levels by facilitating the excretion of excess estrogen from the body. It should be noted that lignans are thought to be estrogen modulators, balancing estrogen activity with both weak estrogenic and anti-estrogenic abilities.

### Pioneering Lignan Research

Use of flaxseed as a cancer prophylactic is "an area that I think has a lot of promise," notes Lilian U. Thompson, Ph.D., of the University of Toronto, one of the world's leading authorities on flax's human health benefits, especially in the area of its use as part of breast cancer prevention and treatment.

Did you know that flaxseed lignans can actually help to shrink tumors in animal studies? Early on, it had been shown that flaxseed lignans are protective at the very early stages of tumor formation when fully developed tumors have not formed, but enough cellular changes were present to indicate the onset of malignancy. Dr. Thompson, however, wanted to know something more: whether supplementation with flaxseed, beginning 13 weeks after carcinogen administration, would reduce the size of already established mammary tumors present—as well as inhibit development of new tumors.[59] In her study, after 7 weeks of treatment, established tumor volume was over 50 percent smaller in all treatment groups, while there was no change in the placebo group. The correlation between established tumor volume and urinary lignan excretion "indicates that the reduction in tumor size is due in part to the lignans derived from…flaxseed."

These findings are confirmed by additional work by Thompson and colleagues, who note that in another experimental study, dietary supplementation with flaxseed or isolated lignans has reduced chemically induced mammary tumor size and number.[60]

There's a lot more to the protective powers of flax lignans. They also seem to weaken the toxic effects of excess estrogen—especially the most potent types of estrogen in women's bodies that are associated with cancerous processes. A woman's cumulative lifetime exposure to estrogen, including the length of her estrous cycle, plays an important role in her lifetime breast cancer risk. The more estrogen to which her tissues are exposed, the greater her risk. Because flax lignans are weakly estrogenic, it has been thought that they might displace more potent forms of estrogen from the receptors of breast cells. These potent forms of estrogen are likely to increase women's risk of cancer. In this sense, because they are weak estrogens, it has been speculated that flax's lignans might have a beneficial anti-estrogenic effect much like the drug tamoxifen—but without its risks.[61]

In fact, the anti-estrogenic effects of flaxseed have been compared with tamoxifen by monitoring estrous cycles. Four-week supplementation of a high-fat diet with flaxseed produced a dose-related cessation or lengthening of the cycle in about two-thirds of animals. With tamoxifen, 83 percent of the animals had irregular cycles. Thus, both compounds were anti-estrogenic; however, flax performed its activities without tamoxifen's tissue toxicity (including uterine cancer risks).

In a 1999 report in *Carcinogenesis,* Thompson and a co-investigator presented intriguing experimental evidence that suggests starting our daughters out on highest lignan content flaxseed oil early on in their lives (including consumption by the mother during pregnancy) can reduce their lifetime breast cancer risk.[62] Flax lignans appear to do so by affecting the highly proliferative terminal end bud structures in the developing mammary gland. Stimulating the terminal ends to develop into alveolar buds and lobules has been suggested to be protective against mammary cancer. In other words, cells mature, becoming quiescent (less excitable with slower reproduction), and are, thus, less likely to become malignant. In this experimental study, early consumption of flax also delayed onset of puberty among rodents. Translated into human health, this would indicate reduced risk of breast cancer by shortening a woman's lifetime estrogen exposure.

Comparative biological research suggests a protective role for lignans against breast cancer. Researchers from the Department of Biological Sciences, Clark Atlanta University, Georgia, compared levels of urinary lignans among cancer-resistant primates with those of humans.[63] It was found that primates consuming their regular food excreted large amounts of the lignan metabolites, enterolactone and enterodiol. When fed a high-fat diet, excretion levels were reduced by more than 90 percent—to a level observed in women with breast cancer. The researchers concluded, "Because non-human primates are particularly resistant to mammary and genital carcinoma on estrogen treatment, the present data suggest that the very high levels of phytoestrogens and lignans as found during exposure to the regular diet may partially account for why these primates are so resistant to hormonal manipulations to induce cancer."

A recent Finnish study examined the association between serum enterolactone and risk of breast cancer in Finnish women.[64] The subjects were participants of the Kuopio Breast Cancer Study that involved 194 breast cancer cases (68 premenopausal and 126 postmenopausal) who entered the study before diagnosis and 208 community-based controls (women without breast cancer). Women with the highest serum enterolactone levels had a 62 percent reduced risk of breast cancer. The reduced risk was seen both among premenopausal and postmenopausal women.

Meanwhile, in another recent clinical study using flax, Joanne Slavin, Ph.D., RD, professor of nutrition at the University of Minnesota at St. Paul, decided to see how flaxseeds fared in the ongoing battle against breast cancer. Slavin and her colleagues gave either no flax, five grams of flaxseed, or ten grams of flaxseed every day for seven weeks to 28 nuns in a convent in Minnesota. All the women were aged 65 years or older. The researchers tested the women's blood for levels of sex hormones and also checked their urine for the breakdown products of estrogen. In the women who ate flaxseed, the concentrations of sex hormones known to be associated with breast cancer were reduced. This result strongly suggests the ability of flaxseeds to reduce breast cancer risk.[65]

Another recent small human study, whose results were presented in December 2000 at the San Antonio Breast Cancer Symposium, shows that ingestion of 25 grams of ground flax meal per day, in women with newly diagnosed postmenopausal estrogen responsive (ER+) breast cancer, decreases biological markers of tumor growth the same amount as the anti-estrogen drug tamoxifen, during the time period between diagnosis and surgery. (Tamoxifen treatment was not compared directly to flax meal in this study and the data are compared from two separate studies).[66]

Although much larger and longer head-to-head clinical trial studies in women are needed, these reports indicate that flax meal is potentially effective as a nutritional means of intervening in ER+ breast cancer.

"Flaxseed is a relatively new contender in the health arena, but it shows a lot of promise in fighting disease—including a possible role in cancer prevention," notes the American Institute for Cancer Research, which sponsored the study.

"Any reduction in the rate of growth is a good indicator," Dr. Thompson says. "If flaxseed produces the same effects as anti-estrogens such as tamoxifen, it has the potential for use in both breast cancer treatment and prevention."

These studies support the work of French researchers who recently found that low levels of ALA predict increased risk of breast cancer.[67] The study was published in the February 2000 issue of the *European Journal of Cancer.* This case-control study conducted in central France was designed to explore whether alpha-linolenic acid inhibits breast cancer, using fatty acid levels in breast adipose (fat) tissue as a biomarker of its intake. Biopsies of breast adipose tissue at the time of diagnosis were obtained from 123 women with invasive non-metastatic breast carcinoma, while 59 women with benign breast disease served as controls. Women with the highest levels of alpha-linolenic acid experienced a 74 percent reduced risk for breast cancer, compared with those women with the lowest intake. According to the researchers, the results suggest "a protective effect of alpha-linolenic acid in the risk of breast cancer."

## FLAX INHIBITS BREAST CANCER SPREAD

Finally, we have convincing human evidence that levels of various fatty acids in adipose breast tissue and the emergence of aggressive metastases are intimately related. Thus, even if you get cancer, regular consumption of flax lignans reduces the risk of metastasis. In a

> ### DID YOU KNOW?
> ### Flax Beneficially Influences
> ### Women's Menstrual Cycles
>
> Women consuming highest lignan content flaxseed oil products generally report a reduction in breast tenderness, bloating, hot flashes and other symptoms related to PMS and menopause.
>
> Lignans in flaxseed also assist in the regulation of women's menstrual cycles. In one study, women consuming lignans in flaxseed did not miss a single cycle, compared to the control group that missed several cycles.[72]

### FYI: Benefits for Women from Highest Lignan Content Flaxseed Oil

- Reduced risk of estrogen-related cancers.
- Reduced risk of metastasis of cancerous tumors.
- Reduced hot flashes.
- Reduced bloating.
- Reduced breast tenderness.
- Regulation of menstrual cycle.
- Improved nail strength.
- Improvement in skin texture and appearance.
- Improvement in hair sheen and appearance.
- Lack of cravings for fat-laden junk foods.

study published in the *British Journal of Cancer,* 121 women patients with an initially localized breast cancer were studied.[68] Their breast adipose tissue was obtained at the time of initial surgery and its fatty acid content analyzed. A low level of alpha-linolenic acid (found predominantly in flax) was strongly associated with the presence of vascular invasion, indicating the cancer was likely to spread. After an average 31 months of follow-up, 21 patients developed metastases. Large tumor size, high cell-division rates, presence of vascular invasion and low levels of alpha-linolenic acid were single factors significantly associated with an increased risk of metastasis. The take-home message from this study is clear: optimal levels of flax and its omega-3 fatty acids can reduce risk of breast cancer spread.

In another report, published in *Lancet,* women with newly diagnosed early breast cancer were interviewed by researchers from the University Department of Surgery, Queen Elizabeth II Medical Center, Perth, Western Australia.[69] These women were interviewed by means of questionnaires, and a 72-hour urine collection and blood sample were taken. The urine samples were assayed for various plant constituents including lignans. After adjustment for age at menarche, parity, alcohol intake,

### Christiane Northrup & Flax

"I've been recommending flaxseeds and flaxseed oil for years," says Christiane Northrup, M.D., one of America's leading experts on women's health. "Flaxseed is the highest known source of anticancer and phytoestrogenic compounds known as lignans—a concentration more than 100 times greater than other lignan-containing foods such as grains, fruits, and vegetables. Lignans are plant substances that get broken down by intestinal bacteria into two main mammalian lignans—enterodiol and enterolactone. These lignans then circulate through the liver and are later excreted in the urine. There are a number of reasons why we all should be interested in incorporating more lignans into our diet. The following are some of the most compelling: Lignans have potent anticancer effects. An impressive number of studies have shown that flaxseed lignans are very potent anticancer agents for both breast and colon cancer because of their ability to modulate the production, availability, and action of hormones produced in our bodies. Lignans are potent phytoestrogens. In women who consume flaxseed oil, studies have shown significant hormonal changes and decreased estradiol levels—alterations similar to those seen with soy isoflavones. This makes flaxseed oil or meal a great choice for women who can't use soy or who simply want another source of phytohormones."

### Flax & Tamoxifen

Research conducted at the Department of Nutritional Sciences, Faculty of Medicine, University of Toronto, Canada, shows that flaxseed and tamoxifen alone or in combination can beneficially influence the course of breast cancer by interfering with various steps of cancer cell adhesion, invasion and migration.[70] When flax lignans and tamoxifen were combined, "a greater inhibitory effect on cell adhesion and invasion was observed than with either compound alone," say the researchers. "It is concluded that lignans and [tamoxifen], alone or in combination, can inhibit the steps involved in the metastasis cascade."

and total fat intake, high excretion of both equol (a plant estrogen) and enterolactone was associated with a "substantial reduction in breast-cancer risk," note the researchers. "There is a substantial reduction in breast-cancer risk among women with a high intake (as measured by excretion) of phyto-oestrogens—particularly the isoflavonic phyto-oestrogen equol and the lignan enterolactone. These findings could be important in the prevention of breast cancer."

## ENDOMETRIAL CANCER

Meanwhile, researchers from the Northern California Cancer Center, Union City, report in the August 6, 2003 issue of the *Journal of the National Cancer Institute* that women with the highest intake of phytoestrogens such as lignans are at lower than normal risk for endometrial cancer.[71] The development of endometrial cancer is largely related to prolonged exposure to unopposed estrogens. Phytoestrogens (i.e., weak estrogens found in plant foods) may have antiestrogenic effects, say these researchers. "Obese postmenopausal women consuming relatively low amounts of phytoestrogens had the highest risk of endometrial cancer," they say.

## PROSTATE CANCER

New research demonstrates that milled flaxseed products with their high lignan content have even greater benefits than previously documented for men who wish to prevent or who are battling prostate cancer. This news should be especially important to all men who are interested in reducing their risk for prostate cancer.

In the latest study from Duke University Medical School, Dr. Wendy Demark-Wahnefried and co-investigators studied the ability of flax to inhibit prostate cancer among 25 men who were awaiting surgical removal of their prostates.[73] These 25 men were told to consume a low-fat diet that they supplemented with three tablespoons of ground flaxseed per day. They simply sprinkled the flaxseed into their cereal or other favorite food.

Reporting in the July 2001 issue of the journal *Urology*, the researchers observed that after an average of only 34 days of supplementation with the flaxseed, the men had lowered cholesterol and testosterone levels and experienced an increase in the number of dead tumor cells, compared to historic controls. Their levels of prostate specific antigen, used to measure malignant activity, also fell. No loss of libido was reported.

Similar observations on the power of flaxseed to aid men in prostate cancer prevention and treatment have been made in Europe at the Oncology Centre, Antwerp, Belgium. Writing in 1999 in the journal *European Urology*, researchers noted that Asian men have much lower incidences of prostate cancer and possibly of benign prostatic hyperplasia (BPH) than their Western counterparts.[74] Vegetarian men also have a lower incidence of prostate cancer than omnivorous males. Both Asian and vegetarian men consume low-fat, high-fiber diets which provide a rich supply of weak dietary plant estrogens. The researchers propose these phytoestrogens are helpful in reducing prostate cancer risk.

In addition to their estrogenic activity, many of these plant compounds can interfere with steroid metabolism and bioavailability, and also modulate the activity of enzymes, such as tyrosine kinase and topoisomerase, which are crucial to the ability of cancer cells to proliferate and spread throughout the body.

Although the researchers cautioned that more studies are necessary, the use of dietary milled flaxseed as a means of reducing risk of prostate cancer appears promising. There are no adverse health effects associated with milled ground flaxseed when used at the dosage of three tablespoons daily, as in the most recent study. Besides, milled flaxseed has so many benefits that go beyond cancer prevention and therapeutics. For more information on flax and prostate cancer, see Chapter 12, Flax and Male Health.

## MELANOMA

Researchers from the Department of Biomedical Sciences, Creighton University School of Medicine, Omaha, Nebraska, investigated the effect of dietary supplementation of flaxseed on experimental melanoma cells.[75] Flaxseed reduced tumor occurrence by up to 63 percent. The addition of flaxseed to the diet also caused a dose-dependent decrease in tumor area and volume, implying that it could be beneficial both in prevention and treatment.

"These results provide the first experimental evidence that flaxseed reduces metastasis and inhibits the growth of the metastatic secondary tumors in animals. It is concluded that flaxseed may be a useful nutritional adjuvant to prevent metastasis in cancer patients."

## COLON CANCER

Most recently, Thompson and other researchers from the Department of Nutritional Sciences, University of Toronto, Ontario, Canada, found that lignans significantly reduced the proliferation of four different types of human colon tumor cell lines, even if they were incubated with various levels of cancer promoters.[76]

In an experimental study, researchers determined whether flax could exert a long-term protective effect against colon cancer, and whether its effect may be, in part, due to its high content of lignans and beneficial influence on the activity of the marker enzyme beta-glucuronidase.[77]

In this study, urinary lignan excretion, an indicator of mammalian lignan production, was significantly increased in the flaxseed groups. Meanwhile, the total activity of beta-glucuronidase, an enzyme produced by colon bacteria, was significantly increased in a dose-dependent manner in the groups consuming flax. Four microadenomas and two polyps were observed in the control group, but none in the treated groups. The total increased activity of beta-glucuronidase was positively correlated with total urinary lignan excretion. The researchers noted, "It is concluded that flaxseed has a colon cancer protective effect...."

## PANCREATIC CANCER

Because a number of polyunsaturated fatty acids have been shown to inhibit the growth of malignant cells in lab experiments, researchers investigated whether fatty acids modify the growth of human pancreatic cancer. To do so, they studied lauric, stearic, palmitic, oleic, linoleic, alpha-linolenic, gamma-linolenic, arachidonic, docosahexaenoic (DHA) and eicosapentaenoic (EPA) acids and the effect of each fatty acid on cell growth.[78]

All the polyunsaturated fatty acids tested had an inhibitory effect, with EPA (found in wild fish and formed from alpha-linolenic acid in flax) being the most potent. Monounsaturated (e.g., olive oil) or saturated fatty acids (found in beef and dairy) were not inhibitory.

"The ability of certain fatty acids to inhibit significantly the growth of three human pancreatic cancer cell lines *in vitro* at concentrations which could be achieved *in vivo* suggests that administration of such fatty acids may be of therapeutic benefit in patients with pancreatic cancer," say the researchers. In this case, wild fish, with its rich source of preformed EPA, may prove to be cancer preventive, with flax exhibiting significant, yet lesser, inhibitory properties.

## PRESCRIPTION FOR CANCER PROTECTION

Thus, you can see, based on the latest research, how neatly a recommendation for consuming flax oil and milled flaxseed fits into a prescription for cancer protection.

We're only at the threshold of knowing the full impact of flaxseed's powers to inhibit and reverse cancers. There is so much to gain from adding flaxseed to your diet daily and by baking with flax. Anyone ready for a flaxseed muffin?

Here are a half-dozen keys to reducing your risk and helping ensure, if you do get cancer, it will be the most easily treated, least invasive:

- Be sure to exercise regularly. It used to be thought that 20 or 30 minutes daily or three times weekly was enough. It isn't. About an hour a day of intensive exercise is important.
- Be sure to consume fiber. Flax is a wonderful fiber. Just 30 to 40 grams daily of a quality ground flax product supplies 24 percent of your daily fiber needs in a mix of soluble and insoluble fibers, as well as significant amounts of omega-3 fatty acids, lignans, phenolic acids and flavonoids, and significant amounts of magnesium.

- Eat "good" fats loaded with omega-3 fatty acids, like those from flax oil, salmon, and herring.
- Bake or purchase flaxseed-based foods such as delicious muffins and use several tablespoons in your favorite fruit smoothies (preferably with antioxidant-rich berries, i.e., blueberries).
- Be sure when you purchase whole flaxseed for your baking needs that the label of your product states that the flax is from cold-milled select flaxseed and that it is 100 percent organic and, therefore, pesticide- and herbicide-free. Such a milling process carefully liberates naturally occurring vitamins, minerals, amino acids, lignans, and phytonutrients without damaging delicate omega-3 fatty acids. Concurrently, the surface area of both soluble and insoluble fibers is greatly increased for maximum benefit.
- Another advantage with flaxseed is that the viscous nature of soluble fibers such as flaxseed mucilage is believed to slow down digestion and absorption of starch, resulting in lower levels of blood glucose, insulin and other endocrine responses.

### FYI: Fighting Cancer with Dr. Johanna Budwig's Anticancer Mix

Dr. Johanna Budwig is recognized worldwide as a pioneer in documenting the healing powers of flax. Here's one of her favorite healing recipes. I'm not sure about how it tastes, but I do hear it has helped a lot of people to survive their cancer. She also maintains this helps the body to absorb the beneficial fatty acids in flaxseed. Be aware that there is no documented scientific verification for this formula. Reports are only anecdotal. But I would like to share Dr. Budwig's ideas and experience as a service to readers—though I also advise you to closely follow your physician's treatments.

[Note: Many people who are allergic to dairy products should avoid or modify this recipe, using a hypo-allergenic substitute for cottage cheese.]

Put in your blender:

    1 cup organic cottage cheese or yogurt (low fat)
    2-5 tablespoons flaxseed oil
    1-3 tablespoons freshly ground flaxseed
    Enough water to make soft
    Pinch of cayenne
    Optional: (Add small amounts of any of the following to taste)
        Garlic
        Red pepper
        Champagne

Make very soft.

Eat some every day.

(Adjust quantities for your taste!)

# CHAPTER SIX

# Healing Mood Disorders

There isn't a person living today whose mood and psychological well-being won't benefit from omega-3 fatty acids. However, persons suffering from depression, alcoholism, attention deficit disorder, impulsive and violent behavior or emotional hostility can particularly benefit by favoring omega-3 fatty acids in their diet. In some of the most amazing research done today, scientists have discovered that the type of fat one consumes is "inextricably linked with your state of mind."[79]

Beyond Prozac® and St. John's wort, omega-3 fatty acids may be a healing elixir for persons suffering from depression, hostility or violent, self-destructive behavior. Yes, no matter whether the depressed person utilizes fluoxetine (Prozac), St. John's wort or other synthetic or natural medicines, one will never truly overcome so many of our most common and destructive mood disorders without adequate intake of omega-3 fatty acids. It may be extraordinary to think, but is truthful to say these essential fats appear to be as important as medical drugs or any other natural medicines when it comes to relieving mood disorders.

The brain is comprised of 77 percent water and 10 to12 percent lipids (fats). However, this isn't the kind of fat found in the area of the abdomen, thighs or buttocks. This is structural fat that forms cell membranes and governs cellular function. What's more, the nerve cells of the brain, in a state of optimal nutrition, are extremely rich in omega-3 fatty acids. In fact, the brain's nerve cells contain five times more omega-3 fatty acids than red blood cells. However, the modern Western diet is severely depleted in omega-3 fatty acids. Thus, the nerve cells of persons with mood disorders may be starved of this essential fat.

## EARLY RESEARCH FINDINGS

Dr. Donald O. Rudin must be given credit for launching the early research into the impact of omega-3 fatty acids on mental health. The former director of the Department of Molecular Biology at Eastern Pennsylvania Psychiatric Institute, Dr. Rudin began working with flaxseed oil in the early 1980s with patients at his clinic. At that time, he performed a clinical trial with 44 patients with various mental disorders. Providing from two to six tablespoons a day of flaxseed oil, he found the results to be astounding. Within two hours of providing some patients the flax oil, he observed that their "mood is improved and depression is lifted."[80]

One patient experienced dramatically improved moods. Dr. Rudin says, "Three days after starting on 6 tablespoons of [flaxseed oil] daily, she developed a marked sense of increased physical energy and unique exuberance." This finding was replicated in varying degrees among most of the patients. By six to eight weeks, most of them were sleeping better, more energetic and less anxious and depressed. Switching the patients to other types of fats (i.e., omega-6 fatty acids which are overly prevalent in the modern American diet) resulted in a return of their symptoms.

## ESSENTIAL FATTY ACIDS FOR ALMOST EVERY COMMON MOOD DISORDER

Could it be that the omega-3 essential fatty acid levels play a role in almost all of our most common mood disorders? The preliminary evidence is convincing. Let's take a closer look.

### Depression

Our first clue comes from epidemiological work that has found the lowest rates of depression worldwide seem to be correlated with the amount of wild fish consumed per capita.[83] Of course, wild fish is one of the prime sources of omega-3 fatty acids. It is also known that depressed patients have very low levels of a type of omega-3 fatty acid known as eicosapentaenoic acid (EPA) in their serum and red blood cells. Cutting edge research has also recently pinpointed among depressed persons marked depletions of omega-3 fatty acids in phospholipid membranes of red blood cells (which are thought to hold similar fatty acid concentrations as in nerve cell membranes).[84,85,86]

### Postpartum Depression

It is known that women have a sixfold increased risk for serious mood disorders following childbirth. This risk generally remains quite high for at least two years.[87] Because breast-feeding women are passing on their essential fatty acids to their newborns, it is quite common for researchers to observe depleted maternal omega-3 fatty acids.

Omega-3 fatty acids are essential to the normal brain development of the newborn, especially during the last three months of pregnancy, when the brain of the unborn baby increases threefold in size. If women neglect to take in enough such essential fatty acids, nature will prioritize the baby's needs at the expense of the mother's, and use nutrients from the mother's own body stores. Modern laboratory testing shows new mothers have only half the normal blood levels of omega-3 fatty acids.[88] Nursing mothers may have even lower levels of essential fatty acids, unless they supplement and eat wisely. No wonder it used to be common practice for women to take cod liver oil during pregnancy! Scientists at the

Mayo Clinic note, "The mental apparatus of the coming generation is developed in [the womb] and the time to begin supplementation is before conception. A normal brain cannot be made without an adequate supply of omega-3 fatty acids, and there may be no later opportunity to repair some effects of an omega-3 fatty acid deficiency once the nervous system is formed."[89]

## Impulsive, Violent Behavior

There are many theories on the link between diet and the environment and antisocial behavior. Genetics and environmental poisoning with lead and other contaminants are influences linked to violent behavior. However, studies indicate that essential fatty acids play a critically important role. One study found that violent criminals have much lower levels of a type of omega-3 fatty acid than persons without a history of violence.[90] "A similar phenomenon has been observed in primates," notes Dr. Simopoulos. "Feeding male monkeys a diet with a high ratio of omega-6 to omega-3 fatty acids (33 to 1) has resulted in more slapping, grappling, pushing, and biting."[91]

In yet another study, normal people given omega-3 fatty acids reduced their hostility level as a result of the stresses of daily life. In this study, Japanese scientists gave either omega-3 fatty acids or placebo to college students. During examination week, students given the natural medicine exhibited much more measured goodwill compared to those students receiving the placebo who scored higher on tests designed to measure hostility.[92]

Finally, persons with a history of violent, impulsive behaviors and those with nonviolent behavior were studied for their levels of docosahexaenoic acid, a member of the omega-3 fatty acid family. Violent persons had significantly higher lifetime violence and hostility ratings and lower concentrations of 5-HIAA than nonviolent subjects, according to research from the Laboratory of Membrane Biochemistry and Biophysics, National Institute on Alcohol Abuse and Alcoholism, Bethesda, Maryland. There may be a correlation between plasma DHA levels and violent behavior.[93]

## Heart Disease and Depression

One reason flax oil is excellent for immediately lowering blood pressure may be due to its ability to help people deal with daily stress, or both of these phenomena may be somehow intertwined. In one study, men with high blood pressure were given extremely tough math and verbal skill tests to perform, with concomitant rises in blood pressure. But when the same men received four tablespoons of flax oil, the rise in their blood pressure was much smaller. These men also experienced reduced levels of triglycerides, total cholesterol, and low-density lipoprotein cholesterol with increases in beneficial high-density lipoprotein cholesterol.[94]

It has also long been known that both depressed and hostile persons are far more likely to die of heart disease. There may be an underlying link between heart disease, depression and hostility that until recently escaped the world's best medical sleuths. Some scientists speculate that depressed, hostile or self-destructive persons are less likely to regularly take their heart medicine, or perhaps it is the overproduction of cortisol and other stress hormones which have a negative effect on circulatory health. Another explanation may well be an underlying deficiency of omega-3 fatty acids which is common to each of these conditions.[95]

## MANY MENTAL DISORDERS IMPROVED

Omega-3 fatty acids can also help in cases of agoraphobia, schizophrenia and bipolar disorder. Just read about some of Dr. Rudin's patients and hear what some have to say…

### Kevin

*Kevin was 32 years old. He stayed home almost all of the time and was diagnosed with agoraphobia, a condition in which certain situations—especially being alone in unfamiliar places—triggers almost unbearable anxiety.*

*Kevin suffered from many other unrelated physical complaints, including very dry skin on his hands and shins, tinnitus, spastic colon, spasms of the esophagus, poor sleep, and fatigue.*

*A psychiatrist at the time prescribed valium. It did not seem to help much at all.*

*That was when he was sent to the offices of Dr. Rudin, the Harvard-educated physician and former director of the Department of Molecular Biology at the Eastern Pennsylvania Psychiatric Institute in Philadelphia. It was during this time that Dr. Rudin began to follow a hunch that something was missing from the average American diet—a special group of fats called the omega-3 fatty acids, which are derived from only a few foods, particularly several species of wild fish and flaxseed.*

*Following some 2$^1$/2 months of taking three tablespoons of flax oil daily, Kevin's physical complaints improved markedly, including the disappearance of his tinnitus, and lessening of his ordinary headaches and migraines. After one year, Kevin's anxiety whenever he left home disappeared.*

### Marta

*Marta was 35 and had been housebound for eight years, suffering severe anxiety attacks once or twice a month. She also suffered from dry skin, dandruff, food allergies, premenstrual syndrome, arthritis, chronic fatigue, and low blood pressure (hypotension). After about one year of supplementation with two tablespoons of flax oil daily, Marta had found that she could leave her home and travel quite extensively without feeling her usual unbearable anxiety. Most of her physical symptoms also improved.*

### Debi

*Suffering from schizophrenia since she was 16, now 26, Debi Erin had gone through many hospitalizations in an effort to help her to overcome the daily visual and auditory hallucinations, intrusive thoughts and bizarre, sometimes violent behavior that she was experiencing. After conventional treatment failed their daughter, her parents sought the help of Dr. Rudin.*

*"I must admit at first the whole idea sounded bizarre," Debi recalls. "Both my mother and I were skeptical. Was this doctor a mad scientist pushing some kind of snake oil? After all the research trials I had been through, surely this was the silliest idea yet.*

*"I tried Dr. Rudin's approach anyway. I took 2 tablespoons of linseed [flaxseed] oil plus a vitamin E sup-*

*plement.... 'Oh well, how could it hurt me?' I said to myself. Thirty minutes later, I noticed how calm I was becoming. The sensation of worms in my nerves and quivering in my muscles diminished considerably. After one week on this simple program, my ten-year psychosis subsided.... I've been free of schizophrenia ever since."*

*Debi has currently completed her college education and is working as a registered nurse.*

These are only a few examples of the dramatic results Dr. Rudin's patients experienced when omega-3 fatty acid-rich flax oil was added to their diets. Could a simple regimen of additional omega-3 fatty acids help persons whom medical science had failed? The answer appears to be *yes*.

## THE F-FILES

This section is called the *F-Files,* because at the time of his work in the early 1980s, Dr. Rudin was working in an area of science that had been almost totally neglected by modern researchers.

Omega-3 fats make up one of the two families of fats, the omega-3s and the omega-6s, that are absolutely essential to human life. Yet, Dr. Rudin knew that the dietary availability of omega-3 fatty acids had declined to only 20 percent of the level found in diets a century ago.

Also, even during the 1980s when his initial pilot study involving 44 patients took place and nutrition was on so many persons' minds, he observed, "Although we live in a time of nutrition consciousness, when everyone is enthusiastic about restoring nutrients to the diet, omega-3—until recently—was virtually ignored."

As a researcher with 35 years of experience, Dr. Rudin suspected that many modern diseases were signs of a new kind of malnutrition—an epidemic affecting Americans.

In other words, in his own way, Dr. Rudin was uncovering an unknown natural phenomenon—the key role that omega-3 fatty acids play in maintaining optimal mental health.

With so many patients at his clinic that simply could not be helped by medical drugs and procedures, the doctor wondered what would happen if the omega-3 fats were restored to their diets. Since Dr. Rudin worked in a clinical setting, he decided to set up a small but representative pilot study, using volunteers suffering from chronic ailments that were not being cured by current conventional treatments. He would add the missing omega-3 oils to their diets and see what happened....

## Hilda

*Hilda was a 43-year-old homemaker and mother who had suffered from unipolar depression for six years. Although lithium helped somewhat, almost uncontrollable violent, murderous thoughts continued to plague her. She suffered from extensive muscle pain, an irritable bowel, and dry, scaly skin—symptoms that often indicate an omega-3 fatty acid deficiency.*

*While maintaining her regular medications, she started on three tablespoons of flaxseed oil daily, and her physical ailments began to lessen within only a few weeks. Around the seventh week, her murderous, violent thoughts began to lift.*

*The sense of calm that pervaded her life was something she hadn't experienced in ages, not since the onset of her psychosis.*

*Around the fourth month, Hilda increased her dosage from three to five tablespoons daily. She went into a mania, the first she ever experienced. Returning to only three tablespoons of flax daily, her mania lifted. "This... demonstrates the need for dosage control," notes Dr. Rudin.*

*By the seventh month, Hilda's dry skin had completely disappeared and, that winter, she did not develop sore, fissured fingers as she had for so long. Her improvements held steady at the time of the conclusion of the study.*

### Ricardo

*Ricardo was a 28-year-old paranoid schizophrenic who, for eight years, had suffered from bizarre thoughts and hallucinations. When he watched world events on television, he was convinced that his thoughts influenced their outcome. When he tried to sleep at night, he suffered through "evening movies," hallucinations that lingered for an hour, and that his medication simply could not control. The paranoia that permeated his mind made being with others almost impossible.*

*Upon taking two to four teaspoons of flax oil daily for a few weeks, the "evening movies" completely stopped, and, over the next few months, his paranoia declined. Anti-psychotic medication still was required, but family members observed that he could enjoy "newfound ease and pleasure in the company of others." Again, dosage is a critical issue. When Ricardo experimented with six to eight teaspoons of flax oil daily, he experienced racing thoughts and feelings that could have led to another psychotic episode. Reducing the dosage brought his condition under reasonable control.*

To be sure, not every patient under Dr. Rudin's care experienced such breakthroughs. But, of the twelve mental patients whom he treated with flax oil, nine experienced nonpsychotic interludes while using the natural medicine. According to Dr. Rudin, "This suggested that improvement was possible on the omega-3 program."

## ABRAM HOFFER, OTHER EXPERTS, CONFIRM RUDIN'S RESULTS

Upon publication of his findings, other doctors began utilizing flax oil as part of their healing protocol for helping patients to regain their mental health. After treating some 26 patients with chronic mental illness for ten years or more, Dr. Abram Hoffer reported on his results.[96] While under conventional therapy, around five percent of schizophrenic patients may experience significant gains in mental health. However, in his small clinical study, by utilizing omega-3 oils in addition to other nutritional supplements, some eighteen patients could go on to function normally in the everyday world; three improved greatly; five moderately; and, one not at all.

Most recently, it has been suggested that omega-3 fatty acids act in a manner similar to that of lithium carbonate and valproate, two effective treatments for bipolar disorder. To test whether the omega-3 fatty acids EPA and DHA (found in some wild fish) could help, researchers conducted a four-month, double-blind, placebo-controlled study, comparing omega-3 fatty acids (9.6 grams per day) versus placebo (olive oil), in addition to usual treatment, in 30 patients with bipolar disorder. The researchers found that the omega-3 fatty acid patient group had a significantly longer period of remission than the placebo group. In addition, for nearly every other outcome measure, the omega-3 fatty acid group performed better than the placebo group.[97]

## THE DOCTOR'S PRESCRIPTION

Clearly, the work of Dr. Rudin opens up new pathways of healing in cases of tragic mental states. Equally clearly, such a program must be undertaken with extreme caution under the care of a qualified mental health professional. As we have seen, dosage with both prescription medication or flaxseed oil is critical if one has an extreme mood disorder. Do not attempt to diagnose yourself. If you have any problems maintaining a positive mood, get a professional diagnosis from an open-minded provider. If necessary, educate that person about the value of omega-3 fatty acids in mental health. And then incorporate them into your diet in moderate doses (one or two tablespoons daily). Clearly, the conventional medical community needs to become more aware of the link between omega-3 fatty acids and mood—and the extreme value of omega-3 fatty acids in mental health.

For most of us who seek to simply improve our mood and mental outlooks, we can safely increase our intake of omega-3 fatty acids, both from wild fish and terrestrial sources. Consider taking lab-tested fish oil capsules or consuming wild fish, particularly rich in these essential fatty acids, two to three times weekly. Such sources include wild Pacific salmon, rainbow trout, sardines, and mackerel.

Also, supplement your diet with flax oil, which provides a different kind of omega-3 fatty acid than wild fish. For convenience, consider taking flax oil capsules and augmenting your regimen by utilizing flaxseed in the recipes from Part III of this book.

### FYI: Conquering Postpartum Depression with Omega-3 Fatty Acids

The tragic recent news reports that postpartum depression drove a Texas mother to slay her five children brings this often-overlooked condition into the spotlight.

The mood disorder "postpartum depression" may be linked to omega-3 and other nutritional deficiencies. Bearing and nursing children puts enormous nutritional demands on mothers' bodies. A new mother must eat a diet that is sufficiently abundant in macronutrients (protein, fats, and complex carbohydrates) and micronutrients (vitamins, minerals, and other nutritional factors) to adequately meet the needs of her hard-working body, as well as that of her child. It is critical that women who are pregnant or lactating receive adequate omega-3 in food or supplements. Yet, many women avoid seafood during pregnancy due to high toxic chemical contamination in many such species.

Because breast-feeding women are passing on their essential fatty acids to their newborns, it is quite common for nursing mothers to deplete their own omega-3 fatty acid stores.

Omega-3 fatty acids are essential to the normal brain development of the newborn, especially during the last three months of pregnancy, when the brain of the unborn baby increases in size threefold. If women neglect to take in enough essential fatty acids, the priorities of Nature will cause the unborn baby to receive these nutrients from the mother's tissues. And these limited supplies still may not be enough to meet baby's needs optimally. Modern laboratory testing shows new mothers have only half the normal blood levels of omega-3 fatty acids.[98] The lesson is clear: all pregnant and nursing women should consider supplementation with flax oil.

# CHAPTER SEVEN

# Omega-3 Fatty Acids for Attention Deficit/Hyperactivity & Related Behavioral Disorders

Attention deficit/hyperactivity disorder can be tragic. I remember recently dear friends who arrived at our home with their son who was diagnosed as suffering from ADHD. He was such a workout for everyone. He was going a million miles an hour, hearing little of what we said, too much in a hurry to eat, too much in a hurry to even listen. It was saddening. And he was going to be a very difficult child for his mother. He was being given methylphenidate (Ritalin®), the most well-known and perhaps most commonly prescribed pharmaceutical drug for attention deficit/hyperactivity disorder (ADHD). Interestingly, his mother was vitally interested in what I had to say with regards to other methods of helping her son. She knew of the side effects of Ritalin and its potential complications. I told her about a number of alternative therapies, including flaxseed and fish oils. I don't know yet how my advice helped her son. I hope it does. I hope that the information in this chapter is utilized by many parents. It isn't that I am blindly set against a drug like Ritalin. But I also know that other viable methods of helping these kids exist, including classical homeopathy. Most recently, the manufacturers of Ritalin, and other interested parties, have come under attack for alleged over-promotion of the drug.

In May 2000, a Dallas law firm filed a lawsuit against the Swiss drug company Novartis AG, which manufacturers Ritalin.[99] The suit seeks class-action status on behalf of people who bought Ritalin for their children. Also named in the suit were the American Psychiatric Association and the advocacy group Children and Adults with Attention-Deficit Hyperactivity Disorder, in Landover, Maryland; both were alleged to have generated concern about the condition while promoting Ritalin and receiving funding from Novartis. Although Novartis has called the lawsuit "without merit" and vowed to "vigorously" defend itself, it is predicted that numerous other suits will soon be filed.

It isn't that drugs such as Ritalin are evil. But, these are, after all, drugs. Doesn't it seem strange—and perhaps even a bit hypocritical—that while America wages its "war against [illegal] drugs" so many children are being placed on drugs that may be legal but also are dangerous to their short- and long-term health? Of course, these drugs help some children. But why are so many kids being medicated? What are the deeper problems that we are failing to deal with?

Ritalin, pemoline (Cylert®), dextroamphetamine (Dexedrine®) and amphetamine (Adderall®) are all stimulants. They are basically legalized "speed." And they do help a number of children, so we can't tell parents never to use them. However, "none of these drugs will cure ADHD," notes Andrew Adesman, M.D.[100]

Still, "when they're effective, they can improve attention, reduce restlessness and foster better relations with peers, parents and teachers," adds Dr. Adesman.

Each of the three stimulant medications has roughly a 75 percent response rate. But when all are used, until one is found to be effective, the response rate is said to be 90 percent.

Still, I do wonder if adding one more drug to childhood is wise.

## OMEGA-3 FATTY ACIDS AND CHILDREN'S BEHAVIOR: PROMISING EVIDENCE FOR A NUTRITIONAL CURE

*Impulsiveness. Inattentiveness. Hyperactivity.* We all know the warning signs that often are the prelude to school officials diagnosing children with ADHD.

### FYI: One-a-Day Ritalin on the Way

Because children often require multiple doses of these medications, and it is difficult to ensure compliance, the drug firm Noven Pharmaceuticals, Inc., of Miami, Florida, is now researching a kids' one-a-day Ritalin, as well as a Ritalin patch.[101]

Meanwhile, Celgene Corp. is working with Novartis to market a highly purified form of Ritalin that is said to be an IQ booster as well. I have reservations (see Ritalin Dangers, below).

### DID YOU KNOW?
### Ritalin Dangers

According to an October 20, 1995 Drug Enforcement Administration bulletin:

- Methylphenidate (MPH), most commonly known as Ritalin, ranks in the top 10 most frequently reported controlled pharmaceuticals stolen from licensed handlers.

- Abuse of MPH can lead to marked tolerance and severe psychic dependence.

- Organized drug trafficking groups in a number of states have utilized various schemes to obtain MPH for resale on the illicit market.

- MPH is abused by diverse segments of the population, from health care professionals and children to street addicts.

- A significant number of children and adolescents are diverting or abusing MPH medication intended for the treatment of ADHD.

- In 1994, a national high school survey (Monitoring the Future) indicated that more seniors in the U.S. abuse Ritalin than are prescribed Ritalin legitimately.

*…Continued on page 70*

Is your child on Ritalin? Do school officials want you to put your child on Ritalin because of his or her poor behavior, lack of concentration, or lack of learning skills?

Although teachers and school officials often are the ones who attempt to diagnose children with ADHD, parents should always make the final decision, in consultation with a professional specializing in this field, as to whether the child should be medicated. It is essential that parents make a decision that is in the child's best short- and long-term interest. For some children, drug therapies may be appropriate. But, for others, drug therapy may lead to potential complications, including increased risk for adult behavioral disorders, drug abuse, criminal activity, and possibly even growth inhibition and cancer (since Ritalin has shown some evidence of carcinogenicity). Drug therapy is the course of last resort when all else has failed. Many contributing factors must be first identified and eliminated beforehand. These include food additives, refined carbohydrates, and food allergies.

You'll want to know about the growing medical evidence that omega-3 fatty acids (especially EPA and DHA) may also help—without the dangerous complications of Ritalin.

There are some key clues to why non-drug remedies may be even more effective.

"ADHD children also tend to have more allergies, eczema, asthma, headaches, stomachaches, ear infections and dry skin than non-ADHD youngsters," notes Dr. Rudin and Clara Felix.[102] (As mentioned, Rudin received his medical degree from Harvard Medical School and from 1957 to 1980 served as the director of the Department of Molecular Biology at the Eastern Pennsylvania Psychiatric Institute, Philadelphia. Felix received her B.S. in nutrition from the University of California, Berkeley. Together, they authored *Omega-3 Oils: A Practical Guide;* see Chapter 1.)

Both Rudin and Felix claim that these problems, including ADHD, are part of a modernization-disease syndrome, which arises from malnutrition centered on an omega-3 fatty acid deficiency.

Their contention is supported by growing evidence. The connection between omega-3 fatty acid deficiency and ADHD has been confirmed by studies in which youngsters with ADHD, when compared

---

...*Continued from page 69*

- Students are giving and selling their medication to classmates who are crushing and snorting the powder like cocaine. In March of 1995, two deaths in Mississippi and Virginia were associated with this activity.

- DAWN statistics on estimated emergency room mentions indicate that there were 271 mentions in 1990, 657 mentions in 1991, 1,044 mentions in 1992 and 725 in 1993 (of which 28 percent to 40 percent were associated with abuse for dependence for psychological effects). The number of mentions for MPH was significantly greater than mentions for Schedule III stimulants (six mentions in 1992 and one mention in 1993 for Schedule III stimulants).

- The U.S. manufactures and consumes five times more MPH than the rest of the world combined.

- MPH aggregate production quota has increased almost sixfold since 1990.

- Ritalin may be cancer-causing.

with non-ADHD children, had much lower blood levels of docosa-hexaenoic acid, an omega-3 fatty acid necessary for normal structure of neurons of the eyes and the cerebral cortex (the brain region that handles higher functions such as reasoning and memory). DHA is obtained directly from wild ocean fish sources or from certain algae, or may be synthesized within the body from the alpha-linolenic acid found in flaxseed (although some children might be genetically unable to form this omega-3, which is why ADHD is one situation where we definitely also want preformed EPA and DHA either from fish oil-type supplements or from specific types of wild fish).

## HOW OMEGA-3 FATTY ACIDS HELP ADHD CHILDREN

All cells throughout the human body are enveloped by membranes composed chiefly of essential fatty acids in the form of phospho-lipids. These play a major role in determining the integrity and flu-idity of cell membranes. What determines the type of phospholipid in the cell membrane is the type of fat consumed. Unfortunately, our children's diets, which may be laden with saturated and unfavorable

> **DID YOU KNOW?**
> **What is ADHD?**
>
> Attention deficit/hyperactivity disorder (ADHD) is a medical term that describes children or adults who are chronically inattentive, uncontrollably impulsive, and hyperactive in a manner inappropriate for mental and chronological age. They often have problems both at home and school. As they grow up they are more likely to drop out of high school and experience patterns of antisocial behavior.

polyunsaturated fats from beef, dairy, and corn oil, interfere with the optimal balance of phospholipids in cell membranes. When the cell membranes are composed of excess saturated fats or omega-6 fatty acids, children may exhibit all of the symptoms of ADHD.

A phospholipid composed of a saturated fat or trans fatty acid differs considerably in structure and function from a phospholipid composed of an essential fatty acid. In addition, there are differences between the structure of an omega-3 oil-balanced membrane and an omega-6-dominant membrane.

Up to 80 percent of the fatty acids in the cerebral cortex of the brain are composed of omega-3 fatty acids. It is thought that the cell is programmed to selectively incorporate the different fatty acids it needs to maintain optimal function, assuming that what the cell needs is in adequate supply from the diet. In actuality, what becomes incorporated into the cell membranes is determined primarily by diet. A diet composed of largely saturated fat, cholesterol, and hydrogenated and trans fatty acids, such as the junk food American diet, is going to lead to membranes which are much less fluid and much more dysfunc-tional in nature compared to the membranes of an individual consuming optimal levels of essential fatty acids. Children with such imbalances are more likely to display aggressive, impulsive, and disruptive behavior, lack desirable attention spans, and are more likely to exhibit antisocial behavior.

"A relative deficiency of essential fatty acids in cellular membranes makes it virtually impossible for the cell membrane to perform its vital functions," says Dr. Murray. "The basic function of the cell membrane is to serve as a selective barrier that regulates the passage of certain materials in and out of the cell. When there is a disturbance of structure or function of the cell membrane, there is a tremendous disruption of homeostasis. This term, homeostasis, refers to the maintenance of static conditions in the internal environment of the cell and, on a larger scale, the human body as a whole. In other words, with a disturbance in cellular membrane structure or function, there is disruption of virtually all cellular processes."

Because the brain is the richest repository of phospholipids in the human body, and accurate nerve cell function is critically dependent on proper membrane fluidity and integrity, it only makes sense that alterations in membrane fluidity could dramatically impact behavior, mood, and mental function, adds Dr. Murray. In addition, studies have shown the biophysical properties, including fluidity of synaptic membranes, directly influences neurotransmitter synthesis, signal transduction, uptake of serotonin and other neurotransmitters, and neurotransmitter binding. All of these factors have been implicated in depression and other psychological disturbances in children.

## SCIENTIFIC EVIDENCE

The omega-3 fatty acids are concentrated in the brain.[103,104] Because of their relative scarceness in the American diet, many children—perhaps a majority of children today—are deficient in omega-3 fatty acids. Learning specialists now believe omega-3 fatty acid deficiency leads to unique symptoms during childhood, including behavioral problems.[105,106]

The evidence is certainly suggestive:

- In 1981, researchers first hypothesized that children with ADHD may have reduced nutritional status of essential fatty acids because they showed greater thirst (a symptom of essential fatty acid deficiency) compared to children without ADHD.[107]
- These results were further confirmed in a 1983 study involving 23 maladjusted children and 20 normal children. Essential fatty acid blood levels in poorly behaved children were significantly lower.[108]
- In 1987, researchers further documented the link between symptoms of an essential fatty acid deficiency and behavioral problems. When they looked at 48 children with ADHD, there was significantly greater thirst, more frequent urination, and more health and learning problems than in children without ADHD.[109] Significantly lower levels of two omega-6 fatty acids and one omega-3 fatty acid (DHA) were found in the subjects with ADHD symptoms.
- In a 1995 study comparing plasma essential fatty acid levels in 53 boys with ADHD to a control group of 43 boys without ADHD, researchers found significantly lower levels of omega-3 fatty acids.[110]
- In the April-May 1996 issue of *Physiology & Behavior*, Laura J. Stevens, of the Department of Foods and Nutrition, Purdue University, and co-investigators, found that boys with lower levels of omega-3 fatty acids in their blood showed more problems with behavior, learning, and health than those with higher levels of total omega-3 fatty acids.[111]
- Also in 1996, researchers from the Department of Psychiatry, Technical University, Faculty of Medicine, Trabzon, Turkey, reported that levels of free fatty acids, as well as zinc, were severalfold lower in ADHD children compared to non-ADHD children.[112] Zinc is a known cofactor for the proper metabolism of essential fatty acids.

- Most recently, researchers performed a study to test the effect of omega-3 fatty acids on intelligence scores among 56 18-month-old children.[113] The children were divided into three groups, one that received DHA, one that received DHA and arachidonic acid, and one that received a formula that did not contain either. All children were enrolled in the study within five days of birth and received one of the three formulas for 17 weeks. The children's overall intelligence and motor skills were tested using the latest Bayley Scales of Infant Development (BSID), the standard for gauging the development of small children. No differences were seen in the Psychomotor Development Index. On the Mental Development Index, which measures memory, ability to solve simple problems and language capabilities, the children in the control group received an average score of 98, slightly below the national average of 100. The DHA group received an average score of 102.4 and the DHA and arachidonic acid group received an average score of 105.1. The children will be tested again in four years to see if the gains continue into early childhood.

## DID YOU KNOW?
### Baby Formulas Deficient in Omega-3 Fatty Acids

It is now well understood that DHA (docosahexaenoic acid), the 22-carbon omega-3 fatty acid, is essential to the healthy development of nervous tissue in infants and children. In healthy, well-nourished adults, the major repository of DHA in the body is the nervous system, including the brain and the neurons of the retina of eye. The importance of omega-3 fatty acids in nervous system growth, development, and functioning has become a central issue in the production of infant formulas. The majority of infant formulas have long been nearly devoid of omega-3 fatty acids, while loaded with omega-6 fatty acids. Infants who receive adequate omega-3 fatty acids score higher on aptitude tests and have better visual acuity. This is one of the reasons that mother's milk is thought to be superior to formula. But this benefit is only available if mother is eating an omega-3-rich diet that allows her to provide her baby with omega-3 fatty acids in utero and in her breast milk. Although omega-3 fatty acids are so important to the growth and development of the fetus/infant, it has been demonstrated that most pregnant and lactating women are often grossly deficient in omega-3—because their diets are devoid of this nutrient. In addition, baby formula manufacturers were prohibited from adding omega-3 fatty acids such as DHA to their products. The Government has strict guidelines for the manufacture and contents of baby formula. Adding DHA would violate these monograph guidelines. Fortunately, these guidelines are in the process of being modified to reflect emerging science. Could it be that this same deficiency of omega-3 fatty acids in the adult diet is linked with congenital or neonatal deficiencies that later manifest as attention deficit disorder?

## THE DOCTOR'S PRESCRIPTION

This is crucial information, especially for parents of children who are diagnosed with ADHD and who are presently being prescribed Ritalin.

"We shouldn't be prescribing medicine simply because that's the easiest way to go," notes Dr. Mark Stein, who runs a University of Chicago clinic for children and adults with the disorder.

While all children with ADHD are not deficient in omega-3 fatty acids, we believe that this may be important for at least a major subset of ADHD children. And omega-3 fatty acids may make a dramatic difference among these children. If your ADHD child is not among these, the omega-3 fatty acids, nevertheless, have many other benefits.

In fact, studies show that children whose treatment program includes only medication and educational and psychological therapy continue to be at high risk for vandalism, petty crime, frequency of alcoholic intoxication, and possession of marijuana. Dietary improvements may be the key to fostering long-term mental health and acceptable behavior.

Parents of ADHD children and ADHD adults who wish to utilize omega-3 fatty acids as a method of modifying their behavior should use both flaxseed oil and wild ocean fish sources of omega-3 fatty acids. Flax provides alpha-linolenic acid, the master or precursor omega-3 fatty acid from which other omega-3 fatty acids are synthesized. The rate of conversion of ALA to EPA and DHA varies, depending on the individual biochemistry of the child. The rate can be optimized by avoiding fried food sources of trans fatty acids that inactivate conversion enzymes, and ensuring adequate intake of vitamins $B_3$, $B_6$, and C, and zinc and magnesium to support enzyme activity. Wild fish or fish oil capsules provide EPA and DHA directly, which appears to be a vital omega-3 fatty acid for modifying behavior of ADHD children and adults.

A combination of flax and wild fish is best, especially since flax can be so easily incorporated into many foods, including salad dressings and even delicious types of desserts.

Although EPA/DHA is available in capsule form and various formulas can be recommended (e.g., Barlean's), many children simply do not comply with taking capsules, and many others refuse to consume wild fish such as salmon, which is rich in omega-3 fatty acids.

Thus, flax, which can be inconspicuously incorporated into children's meals, holds many advantages. (see Recipes, Part III).

We recommend the equivalent of one tablespoon of a high-quality, unrefined flaxseed oil per 100 pounds of body weight.

Nursing mothers may have even lower levels of essential fatty acids, unless they supplement. We recommend that pregnant and nursing women take at least two tablespoons daily of flaxseed oil mixed with yogurt or orange juice, or used as an ingredient in salad dressings. Pregnant women and nursing mothers should also consume safe wild fish (e.g., wild salmon) or take fish oil capsules guaranteed by laboratory analysis to be free from toxic pollutants.

# CHAPTER EIGHT

# Important Help for Diabetics

Diabetes mellitus is a chronic disorder involving carbohydrate, fat, and protein metabolism, and characterized by highly increased levels of sugar in the blood and, subsequently, in the urine. In ancient times, the urine of diabetic patients was described as tasting like honey, sticky to touch, and strongly attracting ants. In diabetes, either the pancreas fails to secrete adequate amounts of insulin (a hormone produced by the beta cells of the islets of Langerhans of the pancreas that enables sugar to be absorbed by the body's cells) or else the body's cells become unresponsive or resistant to insulin. When blood sugar cannot enter cells and instead is left in the blood, this causes the complications associated with diabetes, including increased risk for heart and circulatory disease, stroke, kidney malfunction, blindness, and loss of nerve function.

There is a group of symptoms and signs that is quite indicative of diabetes mellitus:

*Persons with diabetes urinate much more than normal.* Such excessive loss of fluids and high concentration of sugar in the blood cause people to become very thirsty. When people drink sugar-sweetened beverages, they urinate even more and become ever more thirsty.

## DID YOU KNOW?
### "Syndrome X" Afflicts Many Americans

Syndrome X is the name that has been applied by both medical doctors and natural medicine practitioners and researchers to a constellation of symptoms that portend full onset of adult diabetes. The main signs of syndrome X include high levels of insulin in the blood, obesity, elevated cholesterol and triglycerides, high blood pressure, and tissue insulin resistance. Flax oil can help to nip syndrome X before it becomes full-fledged adult-onset diabetes.

## FYI: Two Types of Diabetes

There are two types of diabetes mellitus. Type 1 (juvenile-onset) diabetes is also known as insulin-dependent diabetes mellitus (IDDM) and usually arises in children as a result of the destruction of the insulin-producing pancreatic beta cells by the immune system. Type 2 (adult-onset) diabetes is also known as non-insulin dependent diabetes mellitus (NIDDM). It usually afflicts people past the age of 40. However, due to the rise in obesity in children, there has been an alarming manifestation of type 2 diabetes in juveniles. Whereas symptoms may occur within weeks or months in type 1 diabetes, symptoms may occur only gradually, long after the disease has set in, in people with type 2 diabetes. Only about 10 percent of diabetics are type 1.

Type 1 diabetes is generally associated with damage to the beta cells of the pancreas, thus causing people to require lifelong insulin for the control of their blood sugar levels. This damage may be caused by an autoimmune disorder in which the immune system attacks the body's pancreas. In fact, we now know that about 75 percent of cases of type 1 diabetes are accompanied by the presence of beta-cell antibodies, which are produced by the immune system and mistakenly attack the pancreatic tissues. (Among persons without type 1 diabetes, only about 0.5 to 2.0 percent of the population have beta-cell antibodies.) However, in non-insulin dependent diabetes, the problem is generally that the body's cells have lost their sensitivity to insulin; we find that too often obesity is a prime contributing factor of loss of sensitivity.

For type 1 and type 2 diabetes, dietary and nutritional considerations are critical. In fact, for type 2 diabetics, diet, nutrition and exercise are the major pathways by which a healing response may be initiated within the body.

Clearly, frequency of diabetes is closely associated with diets lacking adequate fiber and containing excessive refined carbohydrates such as refined sugar.[114] Diets that are rich in legumes (beans) and vegetables are especially helpful, both for better sugar control and weight loss.

Because the cells (especially neurons in the central nervous system that depend on sugar to function) are internally deprived of glucose, *fatigue and weakness, accompanied by apathy, are often found in persons with diabetes.* People may not be able to even get up in the morning.

*Tingling may occur in the hands or feet (diabetic neuropathy).*

There may be *reduced resistance to infections* such as boils, urinary tract disorders and vaginal fungal infections because the excess blood sugar interferes with the white blood cell utilization of vitamin C.

## INSULIN RESISTANCE: MAJOR FEATURE OF DIABETES

Anyone who is diabetic, or lives with someone who is, knows that one of the main problems in diabetes, especially in the most commonly occurring type 2 diabetes known as adult onset, is insulin resistance, and also that obesity often accompanies the condition.

In simple terms, the main job of insulin in the human body is to regulate blood glucose or "blood sugar." It also facilitates the entry of amino acids into the cell. This function is truly critical. If blood glucose rises too high, a person becomes at risk for dehydration, coma and possibly death.

After a meal, the rise in blood sugar prompts the pancreas to release insulin into the bloodstream, which causes muscle and fat cells to take up the excess sugar and either use it as fuel or store it in a slightly altered form called glycogen in muscle and as fat in fat cells. When blood sugar levels fall, the pancreas produces another hormone called glucagon that prompts the body to convert the glycogen back into glucose or to form glucose from amino acids.

In a perfect world, this balance between the two hormones—insulin and glucagon—enables the body to maintain blood sugar at optimal levels. Unfortunately, for some 16 million Americans, their body does not respond adequately to insulin and is unable to maintain optimal blood sugar levels.

As a result of insulin resistance, not only do blood sugar levels build up, the pancreas releases excessive amounts of insulin. This combination causes diabetic symptoms. In addition, continuous high levels of glucose can cause an unfavorable, non-enzyme-driven binding of sugar molecules to protein molecules that can have deleterious effects. If glucose is bound to antigens (identification proteins) on the surface of cell membranes, this restructuring of antigens can be very confusing to the immune system, which relies on antigens to distinguish self from non-self. Depending on the nature of the new, inappropriate protein-sugar complex, the immune system can misread antigens, attacking misidentified healthy cells as foreign invaders (auto-immunity) or passively misreading antigens on cancer cells as normal.

## MANY AMERICANS AT RISK FOR SYNDROME X

What's more, many Americans, even if not overtly diabetic, are nevertheless insulin resistant and, therefore, prone to syndrome X. Indeed, virtually everyone who is overweight or suffers high blood pressure also suffers insulin resistance, says Dr. Simopoulos. She estimates, "as many as half of the adults in this country may suffer from some degree of insulin resistance."

## EVIDENCE SUPPORTS ROLE FOR OMEGA-3 FATTY ACIDS

Now there is real hope that a special class of fats, found in a few select foods, can help. Recent new evidence suggests that omega-3 fatty acids like those found in flax and wild fish can have an extremely positive influence on the health of diabetics and prevention of the sugar metabolism condition known as "syndrome X."

## FYI: Typical Foods with Low Glycemic Index

*These foods release sugar into the bloodstream gradually and help persons with diabetes or insulin resistance to stabilize their blood sugar levels.*

- Legumes (lentils, chick peas, split peas, kidney beans, white beans)
- Whole-grain rye bread
- Whole-grain, high-fiber cereals
- Whole-grain pasta
- Oranges
- Organic milk and yogurt
- Brown rice
- Bulgur

Most commonly in the modern American diet, healthy omega-3 fatty acids found in wild ocean fish and flax are supplanted by far greater intake of omega-6 fatty acids prevalent in corn, safflower, cottonseed and sunflower oils and saturated fat in commercial beef, pork, dairy and fried foods.

An interesting Swedish study was published in 1994 reporting the effect of fatty acid nutrition on the development of type 2 diabetes. A group of 1,828 men aged 50 were followed for a period of ten years. During that time, 75 developed NIDDM. The serum lipid profiles of study participants indicated that, relative to those who did not develop diabetes, those who did had higher saturated fat and omega-6 fatty acids with low ALA. The researchers concluded that type 2 diabetes is predictable by high levels of serum omega-6 fatty acids.[115]

A report from the *Annals of the New York Academy of Sciences* shows that experimental diets high in omega-6 fatty acids produce insulin resistance. However, supplementing with omega-3 fatty acids such as those found in flax and fish oil restores insulin sensitivity—even though the diet remains high in other fats.[116]

A second study shows diets rich in omega-6 fatty acids from soybean or safflower oil or saturated fat induce far greater weight gain than diets that emphasize omega-3 fatty acids.[117] Indeed, in this study, all groups consumed equivalent calories and grams of fat, but the difference between a soybean-oil diet and one rich in omega-3 fatty acids was the difference in weight between a 225- and a 150-pound man.

## PROFOUND HUMAN CONSEQUENCES

In Australia, researcher Leonard H. Storlien discovered people with muscle cells low in omega-3 fatty acids and high levels of omega-6 fatty acids were most likely to be both insulin resistant and obese.[118] As the imbalance became more magnified, so did their weight and metabolic problems.

There is hope that dietary changes can enhance the body's insulin sensitivity and reduce the risk for syndrome X complications. In 1997, 55 persons diagnosed with syndrome X were assigned to a diet high in omega-3 fatty acids, particularly from fish. After one year, their insulin sensitivity had improved; they also lost weight, and their blood pressure and triglyceride levels decreased.[119]

A second study of 48 people assigned to either a low-calorie but high-carbohydrate diet or a diet rich in omega-3 fatty acids found dramatic health differences between the two groups. After one year, those consuming low-fat, high-carbohydrate diets had higher glucose levels and reduced insulin sensitivity. Persons consuming the omega-3 fatty acid-rich diet had enhanced insulin sensitivity with lower blood sugar levels, elevated high-density lipoproteins (HDLs, the "good" cholesterol), lower triglycerides and blood pressure. They had significantly reversed syndrome X.[120]

### HOW TO ENHANCE INSULIN SENSITIVITY

One key to enhancing insulin sensitivity and curbing problems related to syndrome X is to consume a diet low in simple, refined carbohydrates (such as those found in sweets, desserts, processed baked and prepared foods) and rich in omega-3 fatty acids from flax and wild fish (see our recipes).

You'll want to emphasize wild ocean fish, green leafy vegetables, highest lignan content flax oil, legumes, whole grains and some nuts such as walnuts. Appropriate nutritional supplements, including chromium and niacin, are also important. Exercise is vital.

### THE DOCTOR'S PRESCRIPTION

Most everyone—particularly persons with diabetes—will benefit from consuming more wild ocean fish such as salmon, as well as from taking one to two tablespoons of highest lignan content flax oil daily.

### FYI: Typical High-Glycemic Foods

*These foods release large amounts of sugar into the bloodstream very quickly and produce sharp rises in blood sugar levels.*

- Soft drinks sweetened with sugar
- White rice
- White bread
- Instant mashed potatoes
- Jams and jellies
- High-sugar cereals
- Corn flakes
- Simple sugars
- Corn chips

# CHAPTER NINE

# Taking Charge of Perimenopause

Premenopause is marked by hormonal fluctuations associated with early menopause-related changes; women usually maintain regular menstrual cycles. *Perimenopause* is the transition between the premenopausal phase and menopause and is characterized by changes in estrogen levels, irregular menstrual cycles, and increased menopausal symptoms.

## ESSENTIAL FATS OFTEN LACKING IN WOMEN'S DIETS

Many women experiencing early signs of menopause or who have premenstrual syndrome symptoms will benefit tremendously from flax therapy. This is because flax provides women in their twenties, thirties and forties with primary nutrients that are often deficient in today's diets: essential fatty acids and natural phytohormones.

Essential fatty acids are required for production of hormones, the absorption of calcium, and assist in absorption of fat-soluble vitamins that nourish our skin, nerves and mucous membranes. These same fats further benefit women's immune, cardiovascular, reproductive and central nervous system health. In addition, they are both transformational and beautifying for women's skin, hair and nails.

Volumes of scientific studies on the omega-3 fatty acids in flax have shown how important these are for women's overall health. Not only has flaxseed oil been shown to relieve depression, fatigue, and allergies, it is a specific healing agent for skin conditions like eczema, psoriasis, acne, and dry skin.

There is also emerging research that suggests highest lignan content flax oil is vital for the prevention of breast cancer, a disease that currently strikes one in eight women. The lignans (found in the flaxseed particulate matter) have the ability to normalize estrogen metabolism and facilitate removal of excess toxic estrogens thought to fuel breast cancer.

These special lignan compounds have many other benefits including ameliorating perimenopausal hot flashes and possessing antioxidant activity.

Beware, not all flax oils are good sources of lignans due to filtration of extracted oil. Be sure your flaxseed oil is non-filtered and unrefined and, therefore, an extremely rich source of flax particulates (high in lignan precursors) which are retained in the oil.

## BEAUTIFUL SKIN WITH FLAX

The human body desperately requires dietary fats—the proper fats—for ultimate skin beauty. But too many women have cut out all fats—and that's dangerous to their beauty quest.

Not surprisingly, up to seven percent of the population suffers from skin conditions such as eczema, which is characterized by chronic itchy, inflamed skin that is dry, red, and scaly. Another two to four percent of people suffer from psoriasis, which is characterized by sharply bordered reddened plaques covered with overlapping silvery scales.[121]

The beauty-enhancing oils (essential fatty acids) from omega-3 fatty acids and other oils (such as borage and evening primrose) are absolutely critical to the vitality and youthfulness of your skin.

Yet, although the skin requires fats and oils, what it doesn't need is excess amounts of saturated fats, partially hydrogenated vegetable oils or other types of highly processed fats used to flavor and texturize convenient fast foods.

Beautiful skin requires the *proper* fats in order to maintain optimal skin cell membrane fatty acids and the proper balance of local tissue hormones called prostaglandins.

## SKIN REQUIRES CONSTANT SUPPLY OF ESSENTIAL FATTY ACIDS

Prostaglandins, which strongly influence skin health, are the body's local chemical messengers, governing many processes, including inflammation. They are not stored in the body, but must be constantly synthesized from essential fatty acids that are taken in from the diet and deposited in cell membranes.

The consequences of an EFA deficiency can be devastating to the skin. When the body lacks EFAs, this deficit leads to an imbalance in prostaglandins and resulting skin problems such as dryness, itching, eczema, scaling, and thinning. What's more, nails may crack, and hair will become discolored and thin.

Psoriasis may be one of the skin's indicators of systemic inflammation. Research from the Department of Dermatology, School of Medicine, University of California, Davis, shows that

### FYI: What Women's Health Expert Christiane Northrup, M.D., Says About Flax

"I've been recommending flaxseeds and flaxseed oil for years. Problem is, for whatever reason, I never took my own advice and got around to actually trying them," says Christiane Northrup, M.D., one of America's leading women's health experts, and editor of the newsletter *Health Wisdom for Women*. "I just didn't make the time to go out and get the seeds plus a coffee grinder that I would reserve solely for grinding flax. Several weeks ago, I was asked if I'd be willing to try an organically grown brand of flaxseed that would come with its own grinder. I said, 'You bet; I've wanted to try this for years!'

"When the flaxseeds and machine arrived, I took them straight to the kitchen and ground up a serving, half of which I added to my daily soy drink and the remainder of which I sprinkled on vanilla yogurt. The taste was nutty and buttery, reminding me of my childhood wheat germ days. In women who consume flaxseed oil, studies have shown significant hormonal changes and decreased estradiol levels—alterations similar to those seen with soy isoflavones. This makes flaxseed oil or meal a great choice for women who can't use soy or who simply want another source of phytohormones."

flax may be particularly beneficial in cases of psoriasis. Arachidonic acid, an omega-6 fatty acid found in cell membranes from omega-6 dietary sources, is turned into another pro-inflammatory chemical, leukotriene $B_4$, which is known to accumulate in the lesions of psoriasis sufferers. Eicosapentaenoic acid (EPA), a major polyunsaturated fatty acid found in fish oil and that the body also produces from the raw materials in flax oil, as well as gamma-linolenic acid (from evening primrose or borage oils), are both potent inhibitors of leukotriene $B_4$ generation.[122] "It seems reasonable, therefore, that adequate dietary supplementation with eicosapentaenoic acid or gamma-linolenic acid may offer a novel and nontoxic approach to suppressing cutaneous inflammatory disorders," notes University of California at Davis researcher Dr. V.A. Ziboh.

Another reason for using flax is that, under the influence of omega-3 oils, the body is far more likely to convert gamma-linolenic acid to favorable prostaglandins.

Meanwhile, flax oil is rich in alpha-linolenic acid, which is ultimately converted to less inflammatory prostaglandins and leukotrienes. Flax's omega-3 fatty acids also inhibit the body's production of inflammation-causing arachidonic acid, the raw material for these pro-inflammatory compounds. Arachidonic acid, together with saturated fat, is usually found in products made from grain-fed livestock animals. Flax favorably inhibits the body's conversion of arachidonic acid to pro-inflammatory prostaglandins.

## THE DOCTOR'S PRESCRIPTION

Women should take one to two tablespoons of flax oil daily. Instead of butter or margarine on bread, try using flax as a spread for its pleasant, nutty taste. Flax can also be spread on foods such as baked potatoes (after cooking, of course). If using flax capsules, generally take six capsules three times daily with meals. Flax may be combined with evening primrose oil for even better results when correcting inflammatory skin conditions. Barleans makes a formula for women called The Essential Woman, which is ideal for perimenopause (see Resources, p. 188).

In addition, two to four tablespoons daily of ground, organic flaxseed will add more beneficial lignans to your diet. A lignan concentrate supplement (such as Brevail® from Lignan Research, LLC) is a useful addition or substitute.

# CHAPTER TEN

# When Calcium Gets Stored in All the Wrong Places

Brittle bone disease or osteoporosis is one of the most common causes of disability in women as they age, often causing disfiguration, hospitalization or surgery via falls and fractures. Most women know that adequate calcium is essential for healthy bones. Some women even know that other minerals and nutrients such as magnesium, silicon and boron, as well as vitamin D, are also essential to healthy bones. But what most don't know is that there is growing evidence that essential fatty acids are super bone protectors. Indeed, what seems to happen, at least in some cases of osteoporosis, is that the body's stores of calcium become inappropriately deposited in other tissues and organs, especially the kidneys and arteries, causing kidney disease and, most commonly, arteriosclerosis (or coronary artery disease). Essential fatty acids seem to be able to correct this tendency of the aging body to store calcium in all the wrong places.

Thus, the interaction between essential fatty acids and calcium metabolism deserves further investigation since it may offer novel approaches to not only the prevention of osteoporosis but also in helping prevent calcification of other vital organs that is associated with osteoporosis and which seems to be responsible for so many related deaths, such as those from kidney disease and coronary artery blockages.

## OMEGA-6 FATTY ACIDS

Linoleic acid (LA) is a fat commonly found in cooking oils (corn, safflower, sunflower). "Many researchers speculate that while the American diet is high in omega-6 fatty acids from vegetable oils, much of this fat is rendered unusable by over-refinement or hydrogenation," notes women's health expert Tori Hudson, N.D. The intake of these oils tends to increase the body's inflammation levels and interferes with the synthesis of other essential fatty acids. So these abundant nutrients may be said to be in bodily overabundance.

Gamma-linolenic acid (GLA) is less commonly found in the everyday diet. It is derived from borage, black currant, and evening primrose oils. The body needs dietary linoleic acid to make gamma-linolenic acid. But, often, its ability to do so is impaired. Thus, many persons benefit from supplements containing gamma-linolenic acid.

## How Essential Fatty Acids Aid Bone Health

According to scientific studies, essential fatty acids:

- Increase calcium absorption from the gut, in part by enhancing the effects of vitamin D.

- Reduce urinary excretion of calcium.

- Increase the amount of calcium deposited in the bone.

- Improve bone strength and stimulate synthesis of bone collagen.

As you know by now, alpha-linolenic acid is the parent compound of all omega-3 fatty acids. It is found in seeds, nuts, whole grains, dark leafy green vegetables, and hemp, but most abundantly in flax oil. Meanwhile, EPA, found concentrated in fish oils, is also widely deficient in the American diet. It can be manufactured from alpha-linolenic acid found in flax.

Interest in essential fatty acids and osteoporosis stems from recent research showing essential fatty acid-deficient animals develop severe osteoporosis coupled with increased deposits of calcium in the kidneys and arteries, thereby indicating that the body's metabolism of this vital mineral is impaired.

"This picture is similar to that seen in osteoporosis in the elderly, where the loss of bone calcium is associated with ectopic calcification of other tissues, particularly the arteries and the kidneys," note Drs. M.C. Kruger and D.F. Horrobin, of the Department of Physiology, University of Pretoria, South Africa.[123]

Indeed, such undesirable calcium deposits may portend another way that essential fatty acids aid women's health. Recent mortality studies indicate that undesired calcification of bodily tissues may be considerably more dangerous than the osteoporosis itself, since the great majority of excess deaths in women with osteoporosis are vascular (i.e., blood clots) and unrelated to fractures or other bone abnormalities.

Drs. Kruger and Horrobin note, "EFAs have now been shown to increase calcium absorption from the gut, in part by enhancing the effects of vitamin D, to reduce urinary excretion of calcium, to increase calcium deposition in bone and improve bone strength and to enhance the synthesis of bone collagen. These desirable actions are associated with reduced ectopic calcification."

## EXPERIMENTAL EVIDENCE

In an experimental study published in 1999, a gamma-linolenic/eicosapentaenoic acid combination increased calcium levels in female rats whose ovaries were removed, compared to rats receiving only placebo.[124] However, when the essential fatty acid combination was added to supplemental estrogen, this enhanced the effect of estrogen on bone calcium. Thus, it is reasonable to speculate that essential fatty acids may make estrogen drugs used by women for maintaining bone mass even more effective.

In another experimental study, supplementation with essential fatty acids has been shown to prevent experimentally induced calcification of the kidneys (nephrocalcinosis).[125] The protective effect was enhanced with the addition of the antioxidant lipoic acid.

We also now know that eicosapentaenoic acid (EPA) and gamma-linolenic acid (GLA) have been reported to have positive effects on bone metabolism in the growing male rat.

## CLINICAL EVIDENCE

Based on such experimental studies, Dr. Kruger set up a pilot study to test the interactions between calcium and eicosapentaenoic acid (EPA) and gamma-linolenic acid (GLA) in humans.[126]

Sixty-five women (with an average age of 79.5 years), taking a background diet low in calcium, were randomly assigned to ingest an eicosapentaenoic acid/gamma-linolenic acid combination or coconut oil placebo capsules; in addition, all of the women received 600 mg per day calcium carbonate.

Markers of bone formation and degradation and bone mineral density (BMD) were measured at the start of the study and at 6, 12, and 18 months. Twenty-one patients continued on the essential fatty acid regimen for a second period of 18 months, after which BMD (at 36 months) was measured.

At 18 months, levels of marker chemicals such as osteocalcin and deoxypyridinoline fell significantly in both groups, indicating a decrease in bone turnover, whereas bone specific alkaline phosphatase rose, indicating beneficial effects of the calcium that was given to all the patients.

In contrast, bone mineral density as measured in the lumbar spinal vertebra and femoral (thighbone) areas showed different effects in the two groups. Over the first 18 months, lumbar spine density remained the same in the treatment group, but decreased 3.2 percent in the placebo group. Femoral bone density increased 1.3 percent in the treatment group, but decreased 2.1 percent in the placebo group.

During the second period of 18 months with all patients now on active treatment, lumbar spine density increased 3.1 percent in patients who remained on active treatment, and 2.3 percent in patients who switched from placebo to active treatment; meanwhile, femoral bone mineral density increased 4.7 percent among persons switched to the active treatment.

"This pilot controlled study suggests that GLA and EPA have beneficial effects on bone in this group of elderly patients, and that they are safe to administer for prolonged periods of time," says Dr. Kruger.

## THE DOCTOR'S PRESCRIPTION

This is good news, indeed, for women concerned about their skeletal health. Supplementing your diet with oils high in gamma-linolenic acid may improve absorption of calcium and enhance calcium content in the bone, while omega-3 fatty acids may improve the blood levels of calcium and help to correct a deficient calcium effect in the bone.

It should be noted that most of the bone mineral density studies done thus far have used pure eicosapentaenoic acid (which is formed in the body from alpha-linolenic acid found in flax or can be taken directly with fish oil capsules).

I recommend flax oil, fish oil, and wild ocean fish as sources of omega-3 fatty acids. However, women who choose to use flax as a source of alpha-linolenic acid should reduce their intake of sunflower, safflower and corn oils as much as possible. These oils interfere with the body's ability to synthesize eicosapentaenoic acid from alpha-linolenic acid.

# CHAPTER ELEVEN

# Flax Benefits Women with Polycystic Ovary Syndrome

Many women blame ovarian cysts for everything from painful periods to infertility. In reality, there are different kinds of ovarian cyst syndromes with which women must deal. One of the most troubling is known as *polycystic ovary syndrome* (PCOS), which is characterized by anovulation (no release of viable eggs from the ovaries), irregular or absent menstrual periods, and hyperandrogenism (elevated serum male hormones testosterone and androstenedione). PCOS is the most common endocrine disorder in women of reproductive age.

Women with this syndrome may complain of abnormal bleeding, infertility, obesity, excess facial hair growth, hair loss, and acne. In addition to the clinical and hormonal changes associated with this condition, enlarged ovaries with an increased number of small follicles (polycystic-appearing ovaries), seen on ultrasound, are characteristic. Although ultrasound reveals that polycystic-appearing ovaries are commonly seen in up to 20 percent of women in the reproductive age range, frank symptoms of polycystic ovary syndrome are estimated to affect only 4 to 10 percent of women in this age range.

Women commonly think of this condition as gynecological because it impairs fertility and can cause irregular periods or no periods at all. But while it is true that, in this condition, the ovaries are known to secrete high levels of "male" hormones (androgens), newer research shows that underlying this hormonal imbalance is yet another: elevated levels of the pancreatic hormone insulin. Thus, a growing body of evidence suggests this syndrome is more of a multifaceted disorder of the endocrine system with gynecological consequences.

## WHAT FACTORS CONTRIBUTE TO PCOS?

Polycystic ovary syndrome has so many manifestations that it brings together a wide range of conventional medical specialties—gynecology, endocrinology, cardiology, pediatrics, and dermatology. Insulin resistance is a common among these patients; and, as one might expect, this feature is more pronounced among obese women. This observation suggests that PCOS and obesity synergistically affect insulin resistance. Insulin resistance leads to increased insulin secretion by the pancreas and hyperinsulinemia.

High insulin levels are caused by diets high in refined sugar and starches, low in micronutrients, and the body's consequential tissue resistance to insulin. The main job of insulin in the human body is to regulate blood glucose or "blood sugar."

After a meal, the body's blood sugar rises, prompting the pancreas to release insulin into the blood-stream, which causes muscle and fat (adipose) cells to take up the excess sugar and either metabolize it or store it as glycogen in muscle tissue, or as fat in fat cells. Unfortunately, for some 16 million Americans, body tissues do not respond adequately to insulin and are unable to help maintain optimal blood sugar levels. As a result, not only do blood sugar levels build up in the blood, the body produces excessive amounts of insulin. This causes syndrome X, a prediabetic syndrome, characterized by obesity, high levels of bad cholesterol and triglycerides, hypertension, and eventually, type 2 diabetes. And now, for some women, we can include polycystic ovary syndrome.

Indeed, there are health care professionals who believe that virtually everyone who is overweight or suffers high blood pressure also suffers insulin resistance. According to Dr. Artemis Simopoulos, author of *The Omega Diet* (HarperCollins, 1999), "as many as half of the adults in this country may suffer from some degree of insulin resistance."

Hyperinsulinemia has been causally linked to all features of PCOS—elevated male hormones, reproductive problems, acne, hirsutism, and metabolic disturbances. If beta cells of the pancreas become exhausted from the long-term workload of producing excess insulin, then insulin insufficiency develops, leading to glucose intolerance and type 2 diabetes. (Some women with PCOS also have alterations in beta cell function.) Moreover, insulin resistance in PCOS may be considered a risk factor for gestational diabetes.[127]

The risk of glucose intolerance among women with PCOS is five to ten times higher than normal and the onset occurs at an earlier age (by the third or fourth decade of life). Obesity, family history of type 2 diabetes, and hyperandrogenism may contribute to elevated diabetes risk in PCOS.[128]

## PCOS, DIABETES, AND OBESITY

Many scientific investigators now think PCOS is actually a kind of diabetes precursor. For example, estimates from Northwestern University in Evanston, Illinois, indicate such patients face a risk of diabetes seven times higher than women who do not have the condition. Naturopathic insight into PCOS is focusing, in part, on the common link connecting PCOS and diabetes—obesity. The contribution obesity makes to type 2 diabetes is well established. The influence of obesity on certain aspects of PCOS may arise from its influence on the control of the ovaries by the pituitary gland and the hypothalamus, the control organs of the endocrine system.

The endocrine system is controlled by the mechanism called "negative feedback." As the level of a hormone from an endocrine gland goes up, the release of the stimulating hormone should decline. For example, follicle stimulating hormone (FSH) stimulates the ovaries to mobilize follicles that will produce and release estrogens; follicles will ripen to the point of releasing an egg cell (ovum) during the ovulation midpoint of the menstrual cycle. As estrogen output goes up, the hypothalamus tells the pituitary to release less FSH. Unfortunately, in obese persons, this well-coordinated feedback relationship is disturbed. Fat (adipose) tissue can produce its own estrogens with the help of the enzyme aromatase (estrogen synthase) in a fashion totally independent of the ovaries and endocrine control. The effect of these "maverick" estrogens is to feed back to the hypothalamus/pituitary control a higher level of estrogens, causing a shutdown of FSH release prematurely, leaving small, underdeveloped ovarian follicles, none of which are ripe enough to release an ovum. This explains why women with PCOS are infertile.

But there is good news. Reducing obesity with diet and exercise can rapidly restore fertility in many of these patients.[129]

## FLAX AND PCOS

Now we have reason to believe that the addition of milled flaxseed and flax oil products to women's diets can be quite helpful in reducing the severity of polycystic ovary syndrome. "Ground flaxseeds are emerging as one of the simplest, most affordable supplemental items women can incorporate into their diets," says naturopathic women's health expert Tori Hudson, N.D. Fascinating new scientific evidence is substantiating this view.

The lingans in flaxseed (mainly SDG) are converted by colon microflora into the mammalian lignans enterolactone and enterodiol. These compounds have the ability to inhibit the enzyme aromatase (estrogen synthase) that manufactures the maverick estrogens out of the abundant supply of male hormones (androgens) that are readily available. Inhibition of this enzyme reduces the inappropriate negative feedback to the endocrine system and helps to restore hypothalamus/pituitary stimulation for ovaries to fully develop follicles leading to normal menstrual cycles and ovulation.

### FYI:
### Flax & Weight Loss

Since polycystic ovary syndrome already may involve obesity, it is important women note that they will not gain weight when they consume flax. According to research, diets rich in omega-6 fatty acids from soybean or safflower oil or saturated fat induce far greater weight gain than diets that emphasize omega-3 fatty acids.[130] Indeed, in one study, all groups consumed equivalent calories and grams of fat, but the difference in weight at the end of the study between a soybean-oil diet and one rich in omega-3 fatty acids was the difference in weight between a 225- and a 150-pound man.

## OMEGA-3 FATTY ACIDS & BLOOD SUGAR

In a recent study published by *Obstetrics & Gynecology*, dietary supplementation with flaxseed was compared to hormone replacement therapy. Daily intake of 40 grams of flaxseed was not only as effective as oral estrogen-progesterone to improve mild menopausal symptoms, its intake also lowered glucose and insulin levels.[131]

In the typical modern America diet, healthy omega-3 fatty acids found in wild fish and flax are supplanted by far greater intake of omega-6 fatty acids prevalent in corn, safflower, cottonseed and sunflower oils and saturated fat in beef, dairy and fried foods.

A report from the *Annals of the New York Academy of Sciences* shows that experimental diets high in omega-6 fatty acids produce insulin resistance. However, supplementing with omega-3 fatty acids, such as those found in flax and fish oil, restores insulin sensitivity—even though the diet remains high in other fats.[132]

In Australia, researcher Leonard H. Storlien discovered people with muscle cells low in omega-3 fatty acids and high levels of omega-6 fatty acids were most likely to be both insulin resistant and obese.[133] As the imbalance became more magnified, so did their weight and metabolic problems.

Israeli Jews suffer from higher rates of obesity and diabetes than Americans even though they consume fewer calories and less fat, explains Dr. Simopoulos. This phenomenon has been called "the Jewish Paradox" and is thought to result from their high consumption of oils rich in omega-6 fatty acids.[134] Indeed, Israeli Jews consume more linoleic acid (one of the omega-6 fatty acids) than any other population group in the world.

There is hope that dietary changes can enhance the body's insulin sensitivity and reduce the risk for polycystic ovary syndrome. In 1997, 55 persons diagnosed with insulin resistance were assigned to a diet high in omega-3 fatty acids. After one year, their insulin sensitivity had improved; they also lost weight, and their blood pressure and triglyceride levels decreased.[135]

A second study of 48 people assigned to either a low-calorie but high-carbohydrate diet or a diet rich in omega-3 fatty acids found dramatic health differences between the two groups. After one year, those consuming low-fat, high-carbohydrate diets had higher glucose levels and reduced insulin sensitivity. Persons consuming the omega-3 fatty acid-rich diet had enhanced insulin sensitivity, elevated high-density lipoproteins (HDLs, the "good" cholesterol), and lower triglycerides and blood pressure. They had significantly reversed syndrome X.[136] As Dr. Simopoulos notes, "When your diet contains a healthy ratio of fatty acids, you have a more normal metabolism and a lower risk of syndrome X, obesity, and diabetes."

There may not be a single nutritional supplement or pharmacological drug today that can offer more benefits relative to polycystic ovary syndrome than flax products.

**THE DOCTOR'S PRESCRIPTION**

Flax is a powerful healing food, and now there is good evidence it will help women suffering from polycystic ovary syndrome. Consume 40 grams of milled flaxseed daily, in addition to one to two tablespoons of flax oil.

# CHAPTER TWELVE

# Flax and Male Health

Researchers have found over the years that a deficiency of omega-3 fatty acids—especially docosahexaenoic acid (DHA)—in sperm cells is one of the biomarkers for impaired male fertility. Increased intake of alpha-linolenic acid, the parent compound of all omega-3 fatty acids (including fish oils), can improve male fertility. Flaxseed oil is the richest known source for alpha-linolenic acid, which is also converted to DHA (although fish oil provides it directly).

Experimental work at the Department of Biochemical Sciences, Scottish Agricultural College, Auchincruive, United Kingdom, investigated the effects of supplementing the diet of male chickens with alpha-linolenic acid or DHA directly on the phospholipid fatty acid composition, motility and fertilizing ability of their sperm.

The birds in the control group received a diet supplemented with soybean oil rich in linoleic acid (18:2n-6) whereas those in the test group were supplemented with flaxseed oil (rich in alpha-linolenic acid) or simply DHA directly. (Enzymes in the body can convert alpha-linolenic acid to DHA.)

According to the researchers, "Supplementation with alpha-linolenic acid significantly enhanced semen fertility at week 39." Interestingly, supplementing the diets with DHA directly did not have the same effect. "The results suggest that the small increase in the proportion of [omega]-3 fatty acids in the sperm phospholipids induced by enriching the diet with alpha-linolenic acid is associated with a significant improvement in semen quality."[137]

A Belgian clinical study demonstrated similar benefits. In this study, alpha-linolenic acid was able to pass through the blood-testis barrier and correct the deficiency of essential fatty acids in sub-fertile men. But fish oil supplementation did not achieve a similar effect. This demonstrates that alpha-linolenic acid has its own unique properties not matched by DHA from fish oil.[138]

## ALA, FLAXSEED OIL & PROSTATE CANCER

Recently, statements have been made that flax oil is a contributor to prostate cancer. In fact, the studies quoted do not cite flax oil but the primary constituent thereof, alpha-linolenic acid. Despite this, ALA has proved to be a powerful anticancer agent in numerous studies of other types of cancer. So, why the confusion?[139]

A close inspection of the studies reveals that ALA has been ruled guilty by association. Take, for example, the following study in the August 1999 issue of *Clinical Biochemistry*. The study, entitled "Comparison of Fatty Acid Profiles in Serum of Patients with Prostate Cancer and Benign Prostatic Hyperplasia," shows the amount of ALA in the blood of the cases represented 0.2 percent of total fatty acids, or approximately 2.65 milligrams. The amount of ALA in the blood of the *controls* represented 0.1 percent of total fatty acids, or approximately 1.32 milligrams. The difference between the cases and controls is a mere 1.33 milligrams. While perhaps statistically significant, the net result of 1.33 mg difference is not physiologically significant, especially in consideration of more dominant fatty acids found in the blood of these men. The saturated fatty acid palmitic acid represented 27.9 percent of total fatty acids in the cases and 26.1 percent in the controls. The difference between the cases and controls is an apparently statistically insignificant 7 percent. However, these percentages represent approximately 766 mg of palmitic acid in the cases and only 345 mg in the controls, a difference of 421 milligrams! While perhaps not statistically significant, the actual milligram difference between the cases and the controls is *physiologically significant*. To summarize, there is only a 1.33-mg difference between the cases and controls with respect to alpha-linolenic acid, as opposed to a 421-mg difference in palmitic acid levels.

All of the *in-vivo* (in living whole organisms, as opposed to isolated tissue) studies to date relating fatty acid ingestion to prostate cancer reveal that the greatest incidence is among men with the highest meat intake, correlated to specific saturated fatty acids, such as palmitic acid. Palmitic acid is a dominant saturated fatty acid in red meat. Even grain-fed livestock supply red meat containing a small amount of ALA. This ALA becomes incorporated into the cells of these animals, along with other fatty acids. We ingest these lipids when we eat red meat. This fact, in combination with the historically low ingestion of omega-3 fatty acids over the last 100 years, is why omnivores actually have higher tissue levels of ALA than vegetarians. Therefore, omnivores with a high-meat diet will have slightly more omega-3s in their tissues than moderate meat eaters and vegetarians. Some have misinterpreted this to associate ALA with prostate cancer risk. Yet, these cases may merely indicate that a diet with high-meat intake, providing a dominance of unhealthful saturated fat, as well as hormones used to accelerate livestock growth, might have adverse effects on prostate health.

The cooking of meat adds another issue to be considered. In the process of cooking meat at high temperatures (for example, broiling or barbecuing), there is a strong possibility that ALA is transformed from its natural cis-isomer to the undesirable trans-isomer. Even conventional medical authorities are looking askance at trans fatty acids. However, the ALA ingested in flaxseed oil, expeller-extracted under low heat or in carefully milled flaxseed, is not damaged in this way. Due to the abundance of unsaturated bonds in EPA and DHA, these fatty acids can also be damaged if their animal food sources (such as wild salmon) are cooked at high temperatures.

There are more global reasons to ponder carefully the conclusions drawn by the studies on ALA and prostate cancer. ALA is the parent compound of the omega-3 family of polyunsaturated fatty acids. In green plants, ALA is found on the membranes of chloroplasts (plant cell organelles containing chlorophyll) and is the principal omega-3 fatty acid of green vegetation (comprising 80 percent of the fatty acids in green leaves). ALA is the foundation source material for EPA and DHA in animals. As the bedrock of the food chain, plants have supported all animal life on the planet since the dawn of time. Herbivores throughout history, from brontosaurus to gray whale to wildebeest, have individually consumed tons of green leaves containing massive amounts of ALA. If ALA is, in the context of whole food sources, problematic relative to inducing cancer in any form, massive numbers of herbivores would have keeled over and died of rampant malignancies in each generation over eons of time. This phenomenon would have threatened the survival of all animal species on Earth. The fact that we have not seen this happening during the time humans have walked the Earth strongly suggests that ALA, in its natural state, is not a cause of cancer. Moreover, it seems unfathomable that the Divine plan of Nature would be so distorted and self-destructive as to allow such a phyto-compound, so essential for the sustenance of all life, to be a major contributor to its termination.

Flax oil is not known to increase the incidence of prostate cancer, and has not been studied in such cases. It has not been clearly demonstrated that ALA, in and of itself, increases prostate cancer incidence. It may be an innocent bystander in the presence of dominant dietary and environmental factors that do increase prostate cancer risk. It is possible that ALA in certain foods, once excessively heated or otherwise damaged, may be harmful in these cases. ALA in flax oil processed under low-heat conditions would not be harmed in this way.

This information goes far to reinforce the recommendation of a plant-based diet; but it does not necessarily implicate alpha-linolenic acid. In fact, there are numerous studies related to the anti-carcinogenic qualities of ALA elsewhere in the body. A human trial demonstrating the beneficial effects of ground flaxseed for existent prostate cancer has already been conducted. What is now needed is a follow-up human trial to determine the effects of flaxseed oil on existent prostate cancer. Such a study would settle the issue.

In the meantime, men concerned about prostate health are advised to optimize hydration, prefer organic food sources, reduce intake of red meat, reduce total fat intake to 20 percent of calories or less, while increasing intake of a broad range of fresh, organic whole plant foods. Be sure to take a high-potency vitamin/mineral supplement with zinc daily and use ground flaxseed (such as Barlean's Forti-Flax) in food preparation. Stay tuned to unfolding revelations about flaxseed, flaxseed oil, ALA, and prostate health.[140,141,142,143,144,145]

### Flax—Your Miracle Medicine
### Startling News:
### SHRINK PROSTATE CANCER WITH FLAX & EXERCISE*

University of California at Los Angeles scientists reported January 14, 2003 that 11 days of daily exercise and a low-fat, high-fiber diet can induce prostate cancer cells to die. This is important news for men with prostate cancer or for those men who desire to remain free from prostate cancer.

* Reprinted from *The Doctors' Prescription for Healthy Living*, 2003:7.6:16-17 (see www.freedompressonline.com)

*...Continued on page 94*

...Continued from page 93

In addition, the new research demonstrates that, once again, our *Healthy Living* recommendation to men to include milled **Barlean's Forti-flax milled flaxseed** in their daily diet is right on target.

## Combination of Exercise & Fiber Kills Cancer Cells

The research, published in the journal *Cancer Causes and Control*, is the first to show that diet and exercise can kill prostate cancer cells.

"You can make changes in a short period of time that have a dramatic impact on your health—in this case, on the growth and death of prostate tumor cells," says R. James Barnard, professor of physiological science at UCLA and study lead investigator.

Barnard and his UCLA colleagues studied two groups of men: 14 obese men, ages 42 to 73, without prostate cancer, who participated in an 11-day diet and exercise program; and 8 men, ages 38 to 74, who have exercised regularly and followed a low-fat, high-fiber diet for more than 14 years.

The researchers collected blood serum samples from the 14 men before they began the 11-day program. The researchers mixed these serum samples in dishes with prostate cancer cells. At the end of the 11-day program, the researchers collected a second set of blood serum samples from the same 14 men, and placed these samples in laboratory dishes with prostate cancer cells.

## Prostate Cancer Cell Death Induced

Among the 14 men at the beginning of their diet and exercise program, fewer than 3 percent of the prostate cancers in the cell culture showed apoptosis (programmed cell death). At the conclusion of the 11-day program, more than 40 percent of these cells were on their way to death, and in the 14-year group of 8 men, more than 50 percent of these cells were on their way to apoptosis, or death.

"That was the finding that made our jaws drop," Barnard said.

In an attempt to understand what might be inducing the apoptosis of the tumor cells, the scientists measured blood serum levels of a hormone called insulinlike growth factor-I (IGF-I). The body needs IGF-I as we age in order to stay fit and healthy and fight the ravages of aging. So, in many ways, IGF-I is essential to our health; yet, paradoxically, excess growth factors such as IGF-I should be eliminated from the bloodstream immediately.

Some, but not all, researchers claim that IGF-I induces cell proliferation. But we think IGF-I is simply a "marker" for a derangement in the body's scavenging proteins that maintain normal levels of a whole set of growth factors. We simply cannot live without growth factors; they have proven anti-aging and tissue repair benefits, so it is foolish to think they do not play a highly beneficial role. Thus, rather than reduce our supply, it is better to simply ensure we transport them away once our body is done utilizing what it can; that's where supplements such as flax are invaluable. In addition, think of IGF-I as a marker for many different types of growth factors that are not being effectively removed and are accumulating in the bloodstream.

In the case of IGF-I, in excess it can also wreak havoc in another way, as it can occupy the same receptor sites on cells as its closely related chemical cousin insulin. If the body's cells cannot utilize insulin or take up glucose, its insulin-producing organ, the pancreas, is stimulated to produce more and more of the hormone. The problem, in fact, might not be due to IGF-I at all, but rather lie in the body's overproduction of insulin. "Insulin is the primary factor that stimulates the liver to produce IGF-I," Barnard said. "In previous research, we have shown that diet and exercise lower the serum insulin level; we suspected that diet and exercise should lower the IGF-I level as well, and we have found that to be true."

High levels of insulin and uncontrolled blood glucose levels are clearly a cancer risk factor, and diabetes is linked to at least nine different cancers (i.e., kidney, liver, biliary tract, pancreas, colon or rectum, prostate, breast, endometrium, and ovary), in addition to all cancers, generally.[146]

Meanwhile, with the most current study, at the end of the 11 days, IGF-I levels for the 14 men had decreased by 20 percent. The 8 men who had followed the diet and exercise program for 14 years had IGF-I levels 55 percent lower than the 14 men had at the start of their diet and exercise program.

## Binding Proteins Remove Excess Growth Factors

While IGF-I floats in the bloodstream, it binds to a protein, insulinlike growth factor binding protein-I (IGFBP-I), which limits the amount of IGF-I that is available to interact with tissue. Higher levels of this binding protein are desirable, causing a drop in free IGF-I levels. (Other growth factors are bound by similar acting binding proteins.)

Over the 11-day program, IGFBP-I levels increased by 53 percent, while in the long-term group of 8 men, IGFBP-I levels were 150 percent higher than the short-term group had at the outset of the program.

"We didn't expect the results would be this dramatic," Barnard said. "We found dramatic changes in both IGF-I and IGFBP-I levels with diet and exercise. The important message is you can change your levels of both IGF-I and IGFBP-I in a very short period of time, and that may have an important impact on your prostate health."

*...Continued on page 96*

...*Continued from page 95*

## The Role of Flax in Prostate Health

Many studies now show that men who consume about 40 grams daily of milled flaxseed have reduced risk for prostate cancer and that clinically detectable prostate cancers, if they do emerge, tend not to spread and are more easily treated.

But this fascinating new line of research at UCLA also helps us to better appreciate one of the ways by which milled flaxseed exerts its powerful protective effects.

For example, in the December 8, 2000 issue of *Cancer Letters*, it was reported that flaxseed and its lignan secoisolariciresinol diglycoside (SDG) inhibit mammary tumor development in rats.[147] Granted, it has been known for some time that flaxseed is a potent and essential protector against both breast and prostate cancers in women and men.

But what you probably didn't know about or appreciate until now is the effect that flaxseed has on plasma IGF-I levels. When rats were exposed to a chemical carcinogen, flaxseed significantly reduced plasma IGF-I concentrations. "The anticancer effect of flaxseed and SDG may be related, in part, to reductions in plasma IGF-I," said the researchers.

Meanwhile in the journal *Nutrition and Cancer*, Canadian researchers from the Department of Nutritional Sciences, Faculty of Medicine, University of Toronto, report similar findings.[148] In their study that showed, once again, flax has significant anticancer potential, they found that IGF-I and epithelial growth factor activity were reduced.

In another report from *Cancer Letters*, researchers state that angiogenesis, the production of a network of blood vessels that nourishes tumors, is important in cancer growth, progression and spread.[149] Vascular endothelial growth factor (VEGF) is one key factor in promotion of cancer angiogenesis, they say. VEGFs are bioactive in the extracellular space where they become available to the endothelial cells. Phytoestrogens such as flax lignans have been shown to alter breast cancer incidence and be cancer-protective in rats, probably because they induce the liver's production of VEGF-binding proteins. "We show that supplementation of 10% flaxseed, the richest source of mammalian lignans, to nude mice with established human breast tumors reduced tumor growth and metastasis. Moreover, flaxseed decreased extracellular levels of VEGF, which may be one mechanistic explanation to the decreased tumor growth and metastasis."

# CHAPTER THIRTEEN

# Arthritis and Other Inflammatory Conditions— A Remedy with Omega-3 Oils

Arthritis is an inflammation of the joints and surrounding tendons and ligaments. Among the oldest known afflictions of human beings, it can affect virtually any joint. According to the National Institutes of Health, arthritis's detrimental effects range from slight pain, stiffness and swelling of the joints to crippling and disability. There are two primary types of arthritis: osteoarthritis and rheumatoid arthritis.

Osteoarthritis is caused by the degeneration of the cartilage tissue in the large, weight-bearing joints of the body—mainly the hips and knees.

Rheumatoid arthritis is thought to be caused by an autoimmune condition in which the body's immune system attacks its own joint tissues. With this condition, joints—most commonly the small joints of the hand—become tender, swollen, and, after years of damage, even deformed. It is not uncommon for an arthritis sufferer to have varying of degrees of both types of arthritis. Regardless of the type, the end result is pain and inflammation at the site of affliction.

This fact has led to the popularity of over-the-counter and prescription medications to combat inflammation, and thus diminish pain. Such medicines as aspirin and nonsteroidal anti-inflammatory drugs (NSAIDs) come with long-term side effects, including a worsening of the arthritic condition. They work by interfering with the enzymes that produce the hormone-like compounds called prostaglandins. But I can suggest another avenue of healing which may be much more safe. This involves the use of omega-3 fatty acids to regulate the body's inflammatory processes. Omega-3 oils have been scientifically proven to be powerful anti-inflammatory agents.

## OMEGA-3 FATTY ACIDS, POWERFUL ANTI-INFLAMMATORY AGENTS

The family of local tissue hormones, prostaglandins, regulates local inflammatory response. If too much of the omega-6 fatty acid called arachidonic acid is located on cell membranes, the enzymes that synthesize prostaglandins will convert arachidonic acid into pro-inflammatory prostaglandins. If instead there is a preponderance of EPA on the cell membranes, the enzymes will convert EPA to non-inflammatory prostaglandins. Thus the non-inflammatory prostaglandins are produced from omega-3 fatty acid dietary sources—seed oils such as flaxseed, or from wild deepwater fish. The high content of omega-3 fatty acids in these sources stimulates the body's production of non-inflammatory prostaglandins.

## NATURAL ALTERNATIVE TO ANTI-INFLAMMATORY MEDICATIONS

Unlike medications that interfere with prostaglandin metabolism, omega-3 oils naturally temper the inflammatory prostaglandins, resulting in a decrease in painful inflammation. The difference between the drug approach and that taken with omega-3 oils is that the oils do not come with the common side effects prevalent to the medications. Flaxseed oil, at around $30.00 a month, is far less expensive than common anti-inflammatory medications—and a whole lot safer and healthier. Not only do the omega-3 oils come without side effects, but they also have been medically proven to benefit as many as 50 other common afflictions. In other words, don't be surprised if you notice other health improvements beyond your expectations. Beyond the power of regulating prostaglandins, omega-3 oils have been found to modulate the immune system, lessening the severity of autoimmune conditions, including rheumatoid arthritis.

There have been many studies to validate the use of essential fatty acids, such as the omega-3 in flaxseed oil and omega-3 oils from wild fish, in arthritic conditions.[150,151,152]

## THE DOCTOR'S PRESCRIPTION

The difference between flax and fish oils is the type of omega-3 they provide. Flax provides omega-3 in the form of alpha-linolenic acid. Wild ocean fish oil supplies omega-3 fatty acids in the form of eicosapentaenoic and docosahexaenoic acids. The types of omega-3 fatty acids in fish oils have a much better record of documentation for enhancing the body's healing response in cases of arthritis. Due to dietary deficiencies in nutrients that assist the enzymes that convert ALA to EPA, as well as trans fatty acids that deactivate those enzymes, the long-term diets of many arthritics have encumbered this conversion. For this reason, I would definitely suggest that consumers use both high-quality lab-tested fish oil capsules and flax oil.

While the causes of arthritis are truly multi-factorial, part of the problem can be identified as a clearly defined omega-3 deficiency. Ingestion of foods such as wild fish and flax oil have been found to increase tissue levels of the valuable omega-3s as well as favorably augment non-inflammatory prostaglandins, averting inflammatory conditions. A practical dietary approach would be to lessen the intake of potentially inflammatory omega-6 oils, as well as grain-fed animal products, and supplement your diet with anti-inflammatory omega-3 oils. An average daily dose of highest lignan content flaxseed oil is one to two tablespoons a day. A daily intake of omega-3 oils from both wild fish and flax will prove to be an important dietary consideration for those suffering from arthritic inflammatory conditions.

# CHAPTER FOURTEEN

# Flax and Asthma

Flaxseed may be one of the best natural medicines today for helping children with asthma to better cope with their condition. Supplementing an asthmatic child's diet with flaxseed or flaxseed oil is not only easy to do for parents; it is one of the most positive, cost-effective and beneficial natural approaches to asthma. In some cases, use of flaxseed may help children to reduce or eliminate their need for asthma medication.

## INCREASES IN PREVALENCE AND DEATHS

Asthma is the leading chronic illness of childhood, is responsible for substantial infant morbidity, and has a significant impact on use of health resources, say researchers from the Department of Pediatrics, University of Washington, and the Center for Health Studies, Group Health Cooperative, Seattle.[153]

Other researchers note that asthma prevalence in children has increased 58 percent since 1980 and that mortality has increased by 78 percent.[154] Interestingly, the burden of the disease is most acute in urban areas and among racial and ethnic minority populations; hospitalization and morbidity rates for non-whites are more than twice those for whites.

Although studies illustrating causal effects between outdoor air pollution and asthma prevalence are scant, air pollution appears to significantly worsen symptoms among children already with the disease. Decreased lung function, bronchial inflammation and other asthma symptoms such as recurrent wheezing, breathlessness, chest tightness and coughing have been associated with exposure to particulates, ozone, smoke, sulfur dioxide, and nitric oxide.

### FYI: Something to Think About: Don't Let Asthma Leave You Breathless

About one of every five athletes who participated in the 1996 Summer Olympic Games in Atlanta had a personal history of asthma, had symptoms that suggested asthma, or took asthma medications, note researchers from the University of Iowa, Iowa City, and the United States Olympic Committee, Colorado Springs, Colorado.[155] This should tell us that when proper steps are taken, children with asthma can go on to achieve great things even in elite sports competition.

## HOW FLAXSEED HELPS

Research in the past decade has revealed the importance of inflammation of the airways in asthma and successful clinical therapies aimed at reducing chronic inflammation. Asthma is associated with the local tissue production of those pro-inflammatory fatty acid metabolites, leukotrienes, which are secreted by the immune system's white blood cells (leukocytes) as a reaction to common environmental allergens and pollutants including house dust mites, animal dander, cockroaches, fungal spores, pollens, and industrial airborne contaminants.

Ordinarily, white blood cells defend the body against infecting organisms and foreign agents, both in the tissues and in the bloodstream itself. But in persons with asthma, the white blood cells tend to produce excess amounts of inflammatory leukotrienes.

One way to counter the body's excess production of undesirable forms of leukotrienes is to enhance intake of omega-3 fatty acids. The omega-3 fatty acids cause cells to produce more non-inflammatory leukotrienes and fewer of those that are prone to increase inflammatory processes. This shift from pro-inflammatory to non-inflammatory leukotrienes is directly related to relief from asthma symptoms, notes a researcher reporting in the *American Journal of Clinical Nutrition*.[156]

Some types of wild fish—such as mackerel and wild Pacific salmon—are a rich source of omega-3 fatty acids, and it has been shown that children who eat fish more than once a week have only one-third the risk of asthma compared with children who do not eat fish regularly.[157]

However, it is often difficult to convince children to consume those wild fish dishes highest in omega-3 fatty acids (e.g., salmon and mackerel) or to take fish oil capsules, including even those that are flavored.

Flaxseed oil can be blended into tasty smoothies, yogurt and spread on bread. What's more, flaxseed also has some pretty good evidence that supports its use in cases of asthma. Recent studies have shown that alpha-linolenic acid, the omega-3 fatty acid found in flaxseed, has a profound ability to inhibit the generation of pro-inflammatory leukotrienes by white blood cells in persons with asthma. Japanese researchers reporting in the *International Archives of Allergy and Immunology* compared the clinical features of patients with asthma who had received a supplemental oil rich in alpha-linolenic acid compared to a group not receiving the nutrient.[158] The scientists found that after only two weeks of supplementation, generation of pro-inflammatory leukotrienes by white blood cells (known as leukocytes) decreased significantly in the intervention group. In contrast, the production of pro-inflammatory leukotrienes "increased significantly" among persons not receiving the alpha-linolenic acid supplement. Even more intriguing, after only four weeks of dietary supplementation, lung function among the intervention group was significantly enhanced by the addition of an alpha-linolenic acid diet. Furthermore, blood levels of total cholesterol, low-density lipoprotein (LDL) cholesterol and triglycerides were significantly decreased by dietary supplementation with the alpha-linolenic acid-rich oil. The researchers concluded that dietary supplementation with alpha-linolenic acid with asthma suppresses the generation of leukotrienes and can have many beneficial therapeutic effects among asthma patients.

In another study conducted by the same scientific team, the effects of alpha-linolenic acid on bronchial asthma were compared with the effects of corn oil for lung function and generation of leukotrienes.[159] (Corn oil, of course, is a commonly consumed vegetable oil that just happens to stimulate the production of pro-inflammatory fatty acids.) In this study, 14 persons with asthma were divided randomly into two equal groups: one consumed alpha-linolenic acid and the other corn oil for four weeks. The generation of pro-inflammatory leukotrienes tended to increase in persons receiving the corn oil and decrease among persons whose diets were supplemented with alpha-linolenic acid. Again, lung function was better among persons receiving the alpha-linolenic acid. These results suggest that alpha-linolenic acid supplementation "is useful for the treatment of asthma in terms of suppression of [pro-inflammatory leukotriene] generation by leucocytes, and improvement of pulmonary function."

In a third study, the effects of eicosapentaenoic acid were studied on asthma symptoms.[160] Both EPA and alpha-linolenic acid are members of the omega-3 fatty acid family. Alpha-linolenic acid is the parent compound of EPA. Persons who ingest alpha-linolenic acid produce EPA as a byproduct of the metabolism of the parent compound—although EPA may be obtained directly from fish oil capsules or wild fish, such as mackerel and salmon. In this study, also from Japan, patients were given EPA (1,800 milligrams per day) and they recorded signs and symptoms in an asthma diary during a two-week observation period. Administration of EPA was associated with improvements in symptoms of asthma and improved lung function. Thus, the researchers conclude that this omega-3 fatty acid "may be useful in patients with asthma…"

## THE DOCTOR'S PRESCRIPTION

Asthma is often thought of as a debilitating childhood disease. It shouldn't be. There are tremendous opportunities to aid children with asthma.

Have your child drink lots of pure water to optimally hydrate respiratory membranes. The brand Penta® is great for this purpose. You can find it at health food stores and some other outlets. This is particularly important in exercise-induced asthma.

Supplementing the asthmatic child's diet with one to two tablespoons of flaxseed oil daily can help to provide the foundation for success. It's easy to put flaxseed oil into your child's diet. Simply mix with yogurt or in a daily smoothie. Consumption of wild fish or fish oil capsules rich in omega-3 fatty acids can also help. By telling your child it will help with his or her condition, the child will be more likely to consume wild fish or take fish oil capsules.

# CHAPTER FIFTEEN

# Therapeutic Use of Flaxseed for Kidney Disease

Flaxseed may be one of your body's best friends if you have kidney disease. A great deal of scientific interest has focused on the ability of flaxseed to halt or slow the progression of kidney disease, as well as ameliorate some of the side effects associated with immunosuppressive drugs used to treat kidney disease.

## KIDNEYS: LITTLE KNOWN BUT VITAL ORGANS

Most of us don't know much about what kinds of functions our kidneys perform, even though life cannot be sustained without them.

Your two kidneys are vital organs, performing many functions to keep your blood clean and chemically balanced. The kidneys remove wastes and extra water from the blood to form urine. Urine flows from the kidneys to the bladder through the ureters.

Your kidneys are bean-shaped organs, each about the size of your fist. They are located near the middle of your back, just inside the bottom of the rib cage. The kidneys are sophisticated reprocessing machines. Every day, your kidneys process about 200 quarts of blood to sift out about two quarts of waste products and extra water.

The wastes in your blood come from the normal metabolism of active tissues and from the food you eat. Your body uses the food for energy and self-repair. After your body has taken what it needs from the food, waste is sent to the blood. If your kidneys did not remove these wastes, the wastes would build up in the blood and damage your body.

The actual filtering occurs in tiny units inside your kidneys called nephrons. Every kidney has about a million nephrons. In the nephron, a glomerulus—which is a tiny blood vessel, or capillary—intertwines with a tiny urine-collecting tube called a tubule. A complicated chemical exchange takes place, as waste materials and water leave your blood and enter your urinary system.

Your kidneys also measure out chemicals like sodium and potassium and release them back to the blood to return to the body. In this way, your kidneys regulate the body's level of these substances.

## YOU CAN'T SING THE SONG IF YOU DON'T KNOW THE WORDS–

### Kidney Disease Quick Definitions

**Albuminuria** (AL-byoo-mih-NOO-ree-uh)—More than normal amounts of a protein called albumin in the urine. Albuminuria may be a sign of kidney disease.

**Creatinine** (kree-AT-ih-nin)—A waste product from meat protein in the diet and from the muscles of the body. Creatinine is removed from blood by the kidneys; as kidney disease progresses, the level of creatinine in the blood increases.

**Polycystic** (PAHL-ee-SIS-tik) **Kidney Disease (PKD)**—An inherited disorder characterized by many grape-like clusters of fluid-filled cysts that make both kidneys larger over time. These cysts take over and destroy working kidney tissue. PKD may cause chronic renal failure and end-stage renal disease.

**Proteinuria** (PRO-tee-NOOR-ee-uh)—The presence of protein in the urine, indicating that the kidney filtration units have been damaged.

## KIDNEY-RELATED DISEASES

Most kidney diseases attack the nephrons, causing them to lose their filtering capacity. Damage to the nephrons may happen quickly, often as the result of injury or poisoning. But most kidney diseases destroy the nephrons slowly and silently. It may take years or even decades for the damage to become apparent.

The two most common causes of kidney disease are diabetes and high blood pressure. If your family has a history of any kind of kidney problems, you may be at risk for kidney disease.

Another cause of kidney disease is lupus, a syndrome that results from several related autoimmune processes. For many years, the prognosis for severe forms of lupus nephritis (lupus-related kidney disease) was miserable.[161] During the late 1950s and 1960s, relatively effective palliative treatments—first with corticosteroids and then cytotoxic drugs—were introduced, which remain the principal treatments 40 years later. Although patient survival and kidney function outcomes have improved over the last four decades, these immunosuppressive regimens are not consistently effective. They often involve what experts call "insidious toxicities."

## FLAX & KIDNEY DISEASE

Flaxseed has demonstrated useful anti-inflammatory and antioxidative properties in a number of animal models and human diseases. Flaxseed may also inhibit sclerosis and formation of scar tissue. In recent years, researchers have been investigating whether the phytoestrogens and lignans from foods such as flaxseed can play a beneficially therapeutic role in kidney disease, which often involves destructive inflammatory, oxidative and sclerotic processes. The answer seems to be quite positive.

"There is growing evidence that dietary phytoestrogens have a beneficial role in chronic renal disease," say Drs. M.T. Velasquez and S.J. Bhathena.[162] They note recent findings suggest, "that consumption of soy-based protein rich in isoflavones and flaxseed rich in lignans retards the development and progression of chronic renal disease. In several animal models of renal disease, both soy protein and flaxseed have been shown to limit or reduce proteinuria and renal pathological lesions associated with progressive renal failure. In studies of human subjects with different types of chronic renal disease, soy protein and flaxseed also appear to moderate proteinuria and preserve renal function."

## SCIENTIFIC STUDIES SUPPORT FLAX'S ROLE IN KIDNEY THERAPEUTICS

In a recent issue of the journal *Lupus,* researchers extracted a lignan precursor from flaxseed to determine if it would exert kidney protective effects similar to the whole flaxseed in the case of experimentally induced aggressive lupus.[163] The study showed that flax lignans were highly protective "in a dose-dependent fashion, by a significant delay in the onset of proteinuria with preservation in glomerular filtration rate and renal size." The study suggests that flax lignans "may have a therapeutic role in lupus nephritis."

In a 1993 study, researchers from the Department of Medicine, University of Western Ontario, London, Canada, investigated whether a diet supplemented with flaxseed, rich in alpha-linolenic acid and plant lignans (the latter, potent platelet-activating factor receptor antagonists) could offer kidney protection in a murine model of lupus nephritis.[164] Tellingly, glomerular filtration rate at 16 weeks was greater in flaxseed-fed mice compared with controls. The onset of proteinuria was delayed by four weeks in the flax-treated mice. The percentage of flaxseed-fed mice with proteinuria was lower than the control mice up to 21 weeks of age. Mortality was lower in the flaxseed-fed mice versus the control mice.

At the Department of Pediatrics and Child Health, University of Manitoba, Winnipeg, Canada, researchers undertook a study to determine if flaxseed would modify the clinical course and renal pathology in experimentally induced polycystic kidney disease.[165] Flaxseed-fed animals had lower serum creatinine, less cystic change, less renal fibrosis, and less macrophage infiltration of the renal interstitium than controls. "Flaxseed ameliorates… rat polycystic kidney disease," the researchers said, by altering the kidney's content of omega-3 fatty acids "in a manner that may promote the formation of less inflammatory classes of renal prostanoids [i.e., inflammatory-mediating chemicals]."

## CLINICAL RESULTS FOR FLAX ALSO PROMISING

In 2001, a clinical trial was conducted to determine whether the kidney-protective effects of ground flaxseed seen in experimental studies would extend to patients with lupus nephritis.[166] Forty patients with lupus nephritis were asked to participate in a randomized crossover trial of flaxseed. Twenty-three agreed and were randomized to receive 30 grams of ground flaxseed daily or control (no placebo) for one year, followed by a twelve-week washout period and the reverse treatment for one year. There were eight drop-outs and, of the fifteen remaining subjects, flaxseed sachet count and serum phospholipid levels indicated only nine were adherent to the flaxseed diet. The nine compliant patients had lower serum creatinine at the end of the two-year study than the seventeen patients who refused to participate. Microalbumin levels demonstrated a greater decline when flaxseed was part of the diet. "Flaxseed appears to be renoprotective in lupus nephritis," the researchers said, but caution that their results could not be construed as definitive.

## THE DOCTOR'S PRESCRIPTION

Most of the clinical trials that have examined the therapeutic role of omega-3 fatty acids and kidney disease were of relatively short duration and involved a small number of patients. Furthermore, it is not clear what chemical constituents in flaxseed are most palliative. Still, the evidence supports the protective effect of flaxseed in a variety of types of chronic kidney disease. In short-term clinical studies, the omega-3 polyunsaturated fatty acids, derived from flaxseed and fish oils, seem to diminish cyclosporine-induced kidney toxicity and the attendant complication of hypertension; to inhibit inflammatory and atherogenic mechanisms in lupus nephritis; and to preserve renal function and reduce proteinuria. But, further investigations are needed to evaluate the long-term effects on renal disease progression in patients with chronic renal failure. If you have kidney disease, discuss the utilization of flaxseed and lignan-rich flax oil for your condition with your health care practitioner and proceed from there.

Particularly in the case of kidney disease, consumers should nutritionally supplement their diet with lignan-rich flaxseed products. Look for flax oil products that specifically state they are lignan-rich. Take one to two tablespoons daily of flaxseed oil, as well as an equal amount of ground flaxseed. Work with your doctor.

# CHAPTER SIXTEEN

# Weight Loss with Flaxseed and Flaxseed Oil

Although classified as fats, omega-3 fatty acids are not utilized by the body in the same way as saturated fats. The omega-3 fatty acid in flaxseed oil does not have the adverse health effects of other fats.

Instead of trying to fool the body with sugar-laden no-fat or low-fat foods, flaxseed, in the context of a responsible diet and judicious exercise, works with the metabolic and physiologic processes of the body resulting in natural weight loss and maintenance. The fatty acids in flaxseed oil have been identified as essential nutrients. This is to say that the body cannot convert other food sources into the essential fatty acids in flaxseed oil. As a result, your body actually craves and looks for these essential nutrients in the foods you eat. If they are not there, the body engages in compensatory mechanisms to survive under the stress of nutritional inadequacy.

### FYI: Flaxing Your Muscles—The Word in the Gym

Besides its use for weight loss, flaxseed oil has received an overwhelming response from the athletic and bodybuilding community. The consensus is that unlike many of the "fad" products on the market, flax oil is here to stay due to its profound health benefits. An article titled "Best of the Best," published in the bodybuilding and health enthusiast magazine *Muscle Media 2000,* claims flaxseed oil as "the hottest idea in bodybuilding" and "a surprising new category of bodybuilding supplements."

- Dan Duchane in his column "Ask the Guru," writing for *Muscle Media 2000,* ranked flaxseed oil as the number one bodybuilding supplement compared to all other available products.

- In an article written by bodybuilding columnist Jay Robb for *Exercise for Men,* he cites the importance of essential fatty acids in flax as primary building blocks of healthy cells; lowering cholesterol levels; forming nerve and brain tissue; playing a key role in regulating the cardiovascular, immune and digestive systems; promoting healing; and, helping to burn calories.

Adding flaxseed oil and ground flaxseed to your foods or taking them with a meal creates a feeling of satiation (feeling of comfortable fullness and satisfaction following a meal). The essential fats in flaxseed oil and the lignans and fiber in ground flaxseed slow stomach emptying. The addition of flax oil and milled flaxseed to food also results in a gradual release of sugar into the small intestine. The physiological effect is a slow, sustained rise in blood sugar, then a prolonged plateau of favorable levels of blood sugar. You will experience a corresponding feeling of prolonged energy, stamina and satisfaction with no hunger pangs soon after the meal. The net result is that you feel fuller longer, and actually eat fewer calories in the long run than if you would have chosen a no- or low-fat diet.

### DID YOU KNOW?
### How Flaxseed Oil Aids Weight Loss

- Decreases cravings for fatty foods and sweets.
- Improves metabolism.
- Creates satiety (feeling of fullness and satisfaction following a meal).
- Regulates blood sugar.
- Regulates insulin levels.
- Increases oxygen utilization.

### THE DOCTOR'S PRESCRIPTION

Dietary fat in and of itself isn't the cause of obesity. Consuming flaxseed oil supports overall metabolism and assures the body it contains essential fatty acids, thus preventing overeating as a compensatory mechanism. The ideal method of taking flaxseed oil for purposes of weight loss or maintenance is in divided doses taken with each meal. Use the recipes in Part III to add flax to your diet.

### DID YOU KNOW?
### Athletes Report These Benefits with Flaxseed Oil

- Enhanced athletic performance.
- Improved stamina and endurance.
- Shortened recovery time from athletic events and strenuous workouts.
- Reliable source of energy without increasing body fat.

- Reduced muscle soreness after strenuous workouts.
- Increased uptake and utilization of oxygen.

# CHAPTER SEVENTEEN

# The Missing Nutrient in Vegetarian Diets

The many health benefits of a well-balanced vegetarian diet have been well documented, including reduced risk of: cardiovascular disease; some types of cancer; osteoporosis; diabetes; and many other conditions. But can a vegetarian diet be improved upon? I say *yes*. In fact, a surprising, newly uncovered nutritional deficiency could be plaguing vegetarians across the country.

Past and present research suggests that vegetarians may be deficient in critical and essential omega-3 fatty acids. Lower proportions of omega-3 fatty acids are found in the blood of vegetarians compared to omnivores (meat and vegetable eaters), note researchers from the Department of Food Science, RMIT University, Melbourne, Victoria, Australia.[167]

In a study by scientists from the Research Institute of Nutrition, Bratislava, Slovakia, the plasma profile of fatty acids was examined in a group of children consisting of 7 vegans, 15 lacto-ovovegetarians and 10 semi-vegetarians.[168] The children were 11 to 15 years old, and the average period of alternative nutrition was 3.4 years. The results were compared with a group of 19 omnivores. Values of omega-3 fatty acids in lacto-ovovegetarians were identical to those of omnivores, whereas they were significantly increased in semi-vegetarians consuming fish twice a week. Due to the total exclusion of animal fats from the diet, vegans had significantly reduced values of omega-3 fatty acids.

The problem seems to be that the major sources of omega-3 fatty acids in the American diet are wild cold water fish such as salmon, sardines, and mackerel, as well as flaxseed. Obviously, wild ocean fish is not an option among vegetarians.

And many vegetarians consume foods very high in omega-3 fatty acid antagonists, such as sunflower and safflower oils, and very little flaxseed. So beneficial are such diets that even with this deficiency, they are excellent for human health among those persons constitutionally amenable to vegetarianism.

However, a diet dominant in omega-6 fatty acids, and all but devoid of omega-3 fatty acids, causes a disproportionate amount of omega-6 fatty acids to accumulate in both animal and human tissues. Recent research all but blames this gross disproportion for the genesis of modern degenerative diseases including arthritis, cancer, heart attack, and stroke. Despite the trace amounts of omega-3 fatty acids present in vegetable foods, vegetarians have also been found to consume more omega-6 fatty acids in proportion to omega-3s than omnivores. This is probably due to the fact that vegetarians consume more omega-6 fatty acid-dominant grains as a staple in their diet than do omnivores.

The lesson here, however, is that while vegetarian diets are great, health-conscious individuals (and what vegetarian isn't aware of his or her health?) can make their diet even better by addressing potential omega-3 fatty acid deficiencies.

Omnivores are also subject to omega-3 fatty acid-deficient diets, but to a slightly lesser extent. Ironically, when livestock are allowed to range free and forage for their food, they ingest vegetable matter containing omega-3 fatty acids. Over time, the omega-3 fatty acids become concentrated in the animals' tissues. When products made from the flesh of these animals are consumed, omnivores unwittingly derive the benefit of the concentrated omega-3 fatty acids in the animal meat. This seeming advantage is becoming less of a factor as animals are kept penned up and grain-fed on demand in order to grow the livestock cheaper and faster and to fatten them for market. Fatty acids in grains are primarily of the omega-6 variety. Omega-6 fatty acids are supplied in the diet at a percentage of 95 percent. Only about 5 percent of our fat intake is omega-3 fatty acids. This is a woeful imbalance.

## HEALTH IMPLICATIONS

In spite of the many benefits to be derived from a vegetarian diet, individual vegetarians may be at higher risk for ailments caused by an omega-3 fatty acid-deficient diet. These include:

- Aching, painful joints and muscles.
- Anovulatory menstrual cycles (i.e., no ovulation).
- Chest pains.
- Cracked nails.
- Depression.
- Dry hair and skin.
- Dry mucous membranes in the mouth, vagina, and other organs.
- Eczema, psoriasis and other skin conditions.
- Fatigue, malaise, lackluster energy, lack of endurance.
- Forgetfulness.
- Frequent colds and influenza.
- Inability to concentrate.
- Indigestion, gas, bloating.
- Irregular heartbeat.
- Lack of motivation.
- Premature wrinkling of skin.

As an example, a recent report in the *American Journal of Clinical Nutrition* found that male vegetarians actually had higher platelet aggregability than male omnivores.[169] In other words, vegetarians were more likely to form blood clots that could trigger heart attack or stroke. Obviously, since vegetarians generally have a lower risk for heart disease or stroke, other facets of the vegetarian diet may minimize this particular negative aspect of circulatory health.

## FYI: Pregnant and Nursing Vegetarian Women Need to Up Their Omega-3 Fatty Acid Intake

This information is critical to women of childbearing age and those who are pregnant.[170] Lower levels of omega-3 fatty acids are also found in the milk of vegetarian mothers as well as the red blood cells of their infants compared to infants of omnivorous mothers or those bottle-fed on cow's milk formula. As a consequence, infants born to vegetarian mothers are likely to have lower stores of omega-3 fatty acids. Due to the importance of omega-3 fatty acids in the development of the nervous system and visual acuity in infants, subtle effects on visual function may occur in the deficient infant.

Omega-3 fatty acids are required for the normal development of the retina and central nervous system, notes Dr. Thomas Sanders, of the Nutrition, Food and Health Research Center, King's College London, United Kingdom. The developing fetus obtains omega-3 fatty acids via selective uptake from the mother's plasma. However, there are greater proportions of omega-6 fatty acids and lower proportions of omega-3 fatty acids in vegetarians compared with omnivores.

Lower concentrations of the omega-3 fatty acid docosahexaenoic acid (DHA) have been observed in blood and artery phospholipids of infants of vegetarians. We know from primate studies that animals with altered or impaired visual function tend to have a high ratio of omega-6 fatty acids to alpha-linolenic acid (the major omega-3 fatty acid in flaxseed oil).

Thus, it is smart to recommend to vegetarian women who are pregnant or nursing diets with a higher intake of omega-3 fatty acids and curbing excessive intakes of omega-6 fatty acids, says Dr. Sanders.

### THE DOCTOR'S PRESCRIPTION

A vegetarian diet has been scientifically proven to prevent and possibly reverse some diseases of modern man. However, due to radical changes in food processing, manufacturing and dietary shifts, vegetarians have been found to be more deficient in essential omega-3 fatty acids than their omnivorous neighbors. This may predispose vegetarians to a variety of health ailments.

The optimal vegetarian diet should include a high quality source of omega-3 fatty acids, such as fresh, unprocessed flaxseed oil, in order to avoid omega-3 fatty acid deficiency and to provide a favorable balance of omega-6 to omega-3 fatty acids in the diet.

An all-natural vegetable source of omega-3 fatty acids may help to prevent and alleviate nutritional deficiency in vegetarians as well as omnivores. The most abundant source of animal-derived omega-3 fatty acids comes from wild cold water ocean fish. The most abundant source of vegetable omega-3 fatty acids comes from flaxseed oil. While it is possible to derive omega-3 in the diet from wild fish or flax, there is a foundational difference between the types of omega-3 fatty acids supplied by each source.

While both sources are excellent, the good news for vegetarians is that the omega-3 fatty acid derived from vegetable sources such as flaxseed oil is a dietary essential. That is, once vegetable omega-3 fatty acid—alpha-linolenic acid—is ingested, the types of omega-3 fatty acids found in wild fish can be formed in the body (as long as trans fatty acids are avoided and the vitamin-mineral cofactors for converting enzymes are sufficient in the diet).

In other words, it is not necessary, in most cases, for vegetarians to resort to consuming animal products to obtain the health benefits of nutritionally required omega-3 fatty acids.

However, vegetarians should lower their intake of omega-6 fatty acids to facilitate the conversion of the vegetable omega-3s to the same omega-3s found in some cold water fish.

The challenge is getting enough essential omega-3 fatty acids required for optimal health. The absolute best choice is unrefined, fresh, organic highest lignan flaxseed oil. Flaxseed oil contains more omega-3 fatty acids than any other common commercial source.

Citing the potential for lower blood lipid levels of omega-3 fatty acids in vegetarians, the American Dietetic Association has advised that, "it is recommended that vegetarians include a good source of ALA in their diet."

The ADA goes on to list flaxseed oil as the richest source of ALA. The high amount of omega-3 fatty acids in flaxseed oil will help to balance out the excessive omega-6 fatty acids prevalent in the American diet.

The recommended dosage of flaxseed oil is from one to two tablespoons a day. However, to receive the most benefit, consumers should make a conscious choice to remove extraneous sources of omega-6 fatty acids from the diet, such as refined foods, common vegetable oils (other than olive) and salad dressings high in omega-6 fatty acids. It would be prudent for vegetarians to use flaxseed oil, which has a very high percentage of omega-3 fatty acids, as the basis for salad dressings, instead of sunflower, corn, safflower, and soy. (See Part III for recipes.)

# CHAPTER EIGHTEEN

# The Smart Flax Shopper

True unrefined nutritional oils are really a perishable food commodity, much like fresh fruit, vegetables, meat and dairy products.

Most nutritional oil companies rely on third-party distributors to stock, inventory and ultimately deliver their products to market, sometimes months after manufacturing. For this reason, most flaxseed oil today is dated for freshness for six months to one year. This is too long for a perishable, electron-rich, easily oxidized, live food like flaxseed oil. What's more, these products are typically shipped by ground transportation resulting in prolonged delivery and conditions such as high heat that may degrade the oil. Worse yet, some companies have resorted to refining and/or filtering their oil in order to artificially extend shelf life.

## CONSUMER BEWARE: 'GLAMORIZING' RANCID OIL

Some manufacturers refine (filter) flaxseed oil to overcome the unpleasant taste when oil turns rancid from peroxidation during long-term unrefrigerated storage. This refining process damages the oil and removes accessory nutrients and antioxidants. Refining causes the oil to become green in color, in contrast to the normal amber color. In order to cover up the green color, these manufacturers add carotenes and vitamin E to restore the natural color. But other nutrients are lost. This nutritional fraud is reminiscent of "enriched" white bread, made from whole wheat robbed of its nutrients, with a few artificial ones thrown into the remaining starch residue to allow the producers to "glamorize" their depleted concoction with the masking word "enriched."

Truly fresh-pressed, organic flaxseed oil has a pleasant, nutty taste and nutritional value which needs no refining.

My favorite brand of flaxseed oil and milled flaxseed is Barleans, of Ferndale, Washington. At Barleans, they are committed to bringing you the absolute freshest oils at their peak of nutritional potency. At Barleans, their oils are made to order, fresh pressed after, not before, they receive store orders. When your local health food store calls in its order for Barlean's flaxseed oil, the oil is pressed that day.

It is then shipped by express air delivery, arriving at your store within a few days of being made. For this reason, Barleans Highest Lignan Content Flax Oil bears freshness dating for only four months for maximum potency and freshness. Because Barleans oils are unfiltered and unrefined, they bring a complete package of lignans, accessory nutrients and antioxidants, just as nature intended.

Ask your friendly vitamin department clerk in your local health food store, and they will tell you that Barleans is the best because it is the freshest flax oil available. Health food stores countrywide have voted Barleans the leading flax oil in the nation year after year.*

## THE MAD FOLKS AT BARLEANS

You might say that at Barleans, they're MAD about fresh flax oil. Here's what I mean:

### Made to Order

At Barleans their flax oil is made to order. They don't make their oil until your local health food store places an order. No inventory or long layovers at distributor warehouses—just great tasting fresh pressed flax oil.

### Air Delivered

Once fresh pressed, they rush their oil by air delivery and manufacturer-direct to your favorite health food store, arriving within just days of being made.

### Dated for Freshness

Each and every bottle of Barleans Highest Lignan Content Flax Oil comes coded with both "fresh pressed" and "freshest before" date stamps spanning a period of four months. Prolonged distributor delivery and warehoused product makes it necessary for other brands to date stamp their oil for six to twelve months. Good for them, not so good for you.

The MAD folks at Barleans call their service **FreshExPress** and it guarantees you the absolute freshest flax

### The Smart Flax Shopper

To obtain high quality flaxseed oil, following these guidelines is crucial. Insist on products:

- Certified by a third party as using organic flaxseeds as raw materials (indicated on label and promotional materials).
- Extracted by mechanical expeller presses only, below 96° F.
- Extracted without the damaging effects of heat, light, and oxygen.
- Packaged in opaque (light resistant) containers.

- Recommended by reputable health and nutrition authorities.
- Delivered manufacturer-direct to retail health food stores.
- Found in the refrigerated section of health food stores.
- Supported with science-based educational materials.

* In fact, Barleans Highest Lignan Content Flax Oil has been voted a five-time Gold Medal Vity Award winner.

oil anywhere. After all, everyone knows that fresh products are naturally better tasting and more nutritious.

## FLAXSEED VS. FLAXSEED OIL

A question often arises concerning the differences between flaxseed and flaxseed oil as components of everyday nutrition. Flax oil is obviously important to support your dietary intake of omega-3 fatty acids because it is a far richer source of omega-3 fatty acids than milled flaxseed. And its uses for salad dressings, smoothies, and as a butter substitute on bread are practical and delicious.

As a proponent of whole foods, I recommend the incorporation of as much of the constituents of flaxseed in the diet as possible. This is why it is generally recommended that consumers take advantage of both oil and milled (ground) flaxseed products. Each has different proportions of various important phytonutrients found in flax and, therefore, unique healthful benefits for consumers. Include ground flaxseed in meal preparation to gain the full benefit of all the nutrients. (Recipes for this purpose in Part III of this book will be helpful.)

Moreover, since we need to counterbalance the overwhelming predominance of omega-6 fatty acids, it is wise to add fresh, unprocessed organic flaxseed oil. Typically, most flax oil is filtered such that lignans are removed from the final product. Prefer fresh, unprocessed flaxseed oil (e.g., Barleans) with high lignan content.

Each health crisis requires intervention tailored to the demands of the patient's individual needs. Therefore, we need to distinguish, as best we can, when it is wise to use a particular form of flax.

Milled flaxseed is your best source of dietary lignans. It is definitely a food of choice for women concerned about breast cancer prevention and men interested in prostate cancer prevention. Flaxseed contains 100 to 800 times more plant lignans than its closest competitors—wheat bran, rye, buckwheat, millet, soybeans, and oats.

Another advantage of milled flaxseed is that it provides relief from constipation. "Flaxseed, like cereals and legumes, has the potential to increase laxation because it provides dietary fiber," notes Artur Klimaszewski, M.D. "There is about 30 grams of dietary fiber in 100 grams of dry flaxseed. This can be especially important for the elderly, who often have chronic difficulties with laxation due to inactivity, low-fiber diets, and/or use of medication for other conditions. In a study of seven subjects whose average age was 78 years, the daily frequency of bowel movements and the number of consecutive days with bowel movements increased among subjects who complied with the dietary regimen of eating 50 grams of flaxseed daily. The flaxseed was provided in muffins and consumed for a period of four weeks."

## DOSAGE

The usual recommendation for adequate intake of dietary alpha-linolenic acid is one tablespoon of flaxseed oil per 100 pounds of body weight, daily. The usual recommendation for milled flaxseed is two to four tablespoons daily.

# CHAPTER NINETEEN

# Flax in a Nutshell

In order for the wealth of information provided in this book to be useful to the reader and consumer, the health-promoting properties of flax must be put into the context of a healthy lifestyle plan that can be followed with relative ease. The recipes that comprise Part III of this book will go a long way in facilitating the addition of fresh, high-quality flax products into your daily routine. Let's look at an overview of how flax fits into a thoroughly designed wellness plan.

The following are what years of experience have taught me are important cornerstones of health and wellness:

- Beneficial genetic inheritance.
- Positive mental attitude, open to new possibilities.
- Loving relationships.
- Optimal intake of pure water.
- Nutrient-dense diet, disciplined to the needs of the body and satisfaction of the palate, thoroughly masticated.
- Judiciously selected nutritional supplements.
- Moderate regular exercise.
- Restful, refreshing sleep.
- Meaningful, self-affirming work.
- Pleasurable hobbies.
- Mind-expanding reading.
- Community service.
- Pollution-free environment.
- Spiritual faith and practice.
- Balanced interaction among all of the above elements with clearly-defined priorities and effective stress-management skills.

Because flax serves as a nutrient source, let's put it into a solid nutritional program. (Be sure to coordinate these recommendations with your health care professional.)

## DRINK COPIOUS AMOUNTS OF PURE WATER

The human body is an entity comprised of water compartmentalized into cells bounded by fatty acids. We must be optimally hydrated for optimal wellness. Do not trust your thirst to tell you when your body needs water. It is unreliable for optimal hydration and declines with age. Drink daily at least the number of fluid ounces equal to half the number of pounds the body weighs. (A 200-pound person should drink twelve eight-ounce cups daily.) As cold temperatures disturb biological processes, drink this water at room temperature or warmer. Minimize intake of artificial beverages, such as soft drinks.

## CONTROL CALORIC INTAKE

Balance caloric intake with physical activity to avoid obesity. Overeating can shorten life span. Dietary self-discipline is essential to longevity. The only factor that has consistently enabled researchers to increase the life span of laboratory animals of all studied species is restriction of caloric intake.

## CONTROL QUALITY AND QUANTITY OF FATS CONSUMED

Emphasize omega-3 sources while reducing omega-6s. Use the recipes provided to add one tablespoon of flaxseed oil to your diet for every 100 pounds of body weight. Control consumption of alcohol, sugar, refined and processed foods, and salt.

## DESIGN A NUTRIENT-DENSE DIET, RICH IN VITAMINS, MINERALS, AND ANTIOXIDANTS

Eat five or more servings of fresh (organic preferred) vegetables and fruits. Prefer vegetables and fruits with brilliant colors indicative of high antioxidant content: dark green leaves, orange/yellow vegetables, purple/blue fruits and vegetables. Let your meal plate be a rainbow of naturally bright-colored nourishment.

Consume six or more servings of fiber-rich whole grains, legumes (beans), and root vegetables (carrots, beets). Add one or two tablespoons of ground flaxseed to daily intake via incorporation into recipes or as an ingredient in smoothies.

Tantalize your palate by mastering the art of using fresh herbs and spices to add culinary excitement and adventure to your eating. It is not an absolute that healthy eating has to be bland and boring. Those who think so just have not explored what is possible with the wide range of natural ingredients readily available in health food stores, groceries, and supermarkets.

## SUPPLEMENT YOUR DIET FOR OPTIMAL MICRO-NUTRITION

- High-potency vitamin-mineral supplement.
- Additional antioxidants (critical to the protection of omega-3 fatty acids on cell membranes).
- Vitamin E: 400-800 IU daily.
- Vitamin C: 500 to 1,000 mg daily.
- Multiple antioxidant formula including botanical antioxidants.

This is the kind of program your body will get excited about. It will reward you with increased vitality and sense of well-being.

# Part III–
# Flax Recipes

# CHAPTER TWENTY

# Flaxseed…Ancient Grain— Designer Food Ingredient of the Future

Flaxseed was once a staple food source used by the ancient Greeks, Romans and Egyptians, supplying ample amounts of valuable essential fatty acids, amino acids, protein, dietary fiber and cancer preventing phytonutrients. Unfortunately, within the last 100 years, modern methods of food processing, combined with preferences for wheat and other less nutritious enriched grain products, have removed many of these essential and vital nutrients from our food chain.

Nutrition research on flaxseed has confirmed its potential as a new (actually ancient) ingredient for breads, buns, and other bakery products. Ground flaxseed (flaxseed flour) can be added to almost any baked product and adds a nutty flavor to bread, waffles, pancakes, and other products if it composes a minimum of six to eight percent of the dry ingredient of the recipe or formula. Some other food uses for ground flaxseed include, but are not limited to, fiber and nutrition bars, protein powders, pastries, pastas, bagels, muffins, crackers, cookies, and cereals, as well as soup and bakery mixes. When partially defatted flaxseed flour is used in baked products, the oil in the recipe can be reduced by the amount of the oil in the added flaxseed (which is usually approximately 10 percent). Gluten content should be balanced in yeast-leavened products. Flaxseed is approved by the Food and Drug Administration for inclusion in foods.

## Nutritional Properties of Partially Defatted Flax Flour

- Ten percent oil, of which 55 percent is essential omega-3 fatty acids (alpha-linolenic acid).
- Valuable source of dietary protein (26 to 28 percent content).
- Rich source of phytonutrients (e.g., lignans).
- Valuable source of essential fatty acids.
- Valuable source of essential amino acids.
- Comprised of 30 percent unrefined complex carbohydrates.
- Valuable source of essential minerals.
- High in dietary fiber, 30 percent insoluble and 10 percent soluble. The latter includes mucilage/gum.

# Put the Fat Back

Put the fat back?

That's right, you read it correctly the first time, "Put the fat back."

I'm sure most of you have heard about good cholesterol and bad cholesterol. Well, guess what? The same is true of fat. In fact, the good or right fats and oils help build the HDL "good" cholesterol while the bad or wrong fats contribute to the LDL "bad" cholesterol.

Did you know that the right kinds of fat are actually essential to life itself, and without them we are much more susceptible to disease and death? What if I told you that the right fats, or more specifically what are known as *essential fatty acids*, protect us from the most devastating diseases of our time, including heart disease, cancer, and stroke? Now, don't take my word for it, research scientists worldwide are rediscovering the almost unbelievable health-enhancing and therapeutic potential of essential fatty acids.

We must learn how to avoid the unhealthy fats such as excess saturated fats from animal foods and the fats from hydrogenated sources like margarine, shortening, and fried foods. Plus, we need to include the vital essential fatty acids from unrefined vegetable oils in our everyday diet.

And this is what this recipe section is all about, putting the right fat into the diet.

You may be wondering about all the no-fat and low-fat food products lining our grocery store shelves. Let me ask you a question. Have you actually lost any weight since going low fat? If you are like most Americans, probably not. In fact, statistics tell us that since America has been cutting the fat, we have actually gained more weight per capita as a nation.

It shouldn't come as any surprise that many of these no-fat and low-fat products are made up primarily of simple carbohydrates from white sugar and/or white flour. Read any label of those fat-free cookies and you will find sugar and corn syrup heading the ingredient parade. Refined carbohydrates have zero nutritional value but are loaded with calories. When eaten in large quantities, they are converted to fat in the body. We are now being served gigantic portions. For example, muffins have become mammoth and bagels have become oversized since the advent of the fat-free era.

Ironically, the fat you have been trying to avoid can actually aid in weight loss if it is the right kind. The essential fatty acids help to adjust metabolism naturally, increasing the body's ability to burn excess calories. The good fats even go so far as to ferry the bad fats out of our cells and tissues. Since bad fats can harbor toxins, this is terrific news all the way around.

Where can we find these so-called good fats—the essential fatty acids? If you lived approximately 100 years ago, you could have found these healthy fats in raw seeds and nuts as well as in vegetable oils extracted the old-fashioned way. Even meats had higher tissue levels of essential fatty acids 100 years ago because animals were allowed to range free and graze on vegetable matter containing the essential fats. These healing and protective fatty acids used to be prevalent in our diets.

Unfortunately, because of modern manufacturing methods and refinement of foods rich in the protective and healing essential fatty acids, these good fats are almost nonexistent in our daily foods. Is it any coincidence that heart disease, cancer, and stroke have become our nation's leading killers since the advent of modern technology for processing foods and oils?

For the first time in almost 100 years, the essential fatty acids are once again becoming available as found in nature's richest source, unrefined flax oil. Thus the title of this book: *The Healing Power of Flax*. People across the country are flocking to their local health food stores for a bottle of this liquid gold.

Dramatic evidence suggests that flax oil, and a special plant fiber found in flaxseed called *lignan*, can protect us against heart disease and cancer as well as other degenerative diseases. For nearly 50 years, Dr. Johanna Budwig, a German biochemist and Nobel Prize nominee, has utilized unrefined flax oil in conjunction with an organic diet to fight cancer. Even here in the U.S., numerous research studies have been concluded with flaxseed and cancer, including research by the National Cancer Institute (NCI). The NCI found that flaxseed did indeed have an anticancer effect—even to match some chemotherapeutic drugs—but without the nasty side effects found with the drugs!

Women have become increasingly aware of the rising epidemic of breast cancer. Unfortunately, one out of eight women today will be diagnosed with breast cancer. Is it possible that flax oil could significantly reduce the incidence of this deadly disease? Scientific research on women and breast cancer has established that women who have the highest amount of the omega-3 fatty acid, most prevalent in flax oil, have the lowest incidence of breast cancer. More important, if any of these women had an existing tumor, those with the highest amount of omega-3 in their breast tissue still had the lowest incidence of the tumor spreading to other tissues and organs.

What about other women's health concerns? The use of flax oil has been found to ease the mood swings and uncomfortable cramping associated with PMS as well as ease the transition of menopause. Also, the essential fatty acids found in flax oil are unsurpassed for building strong nails, lustrous hair, and radiant skin.

If you own a pet, remember to add a teaspoon or two of flax oil to your animal's food. In Europe, flax oil was once widely used to promote beautiful and glistening fur, strong hooves and nails, vibrant eyes, and robust health.

We can all appreciate the added protection against cancer that flax oil can bring, but what about heart disease? Doesn't fat increase one's chances of cardiovascular complications? The answer is yes, and no.

Once again we must qualify the type of fat we are talking about. Excessive ingestion of saturated fat and especially "funny fats" (hydrogenated oils) will increase the likelihood of heart disease, but the absolute opposite is true of the essential fats found in flax oil. Flax oil has been found to significantly decrease the possibility of heart disease on many fronts. Flax oil lubricates and relaxes our blood vessels, helps to clear clogged arteries, and acts as a valuable energy source that keeps the heart beating healthy and strong. This is the reason why flax oil is considered so "heart smart."

The good fats found in flax affect our health at nearly every level. They combat infection and allergy by boosting our immune system. They act as cellular batteries, supercharging every one of our one hundred trillion cells, becoming incorporated into their membranes, and capturing photon energy from the sun.

Now, if I called you a "fat head" you would probably be offended. Yet, it just might be the highest compliment I could pay you. The essential fats found in flax have been postulated to improve memory, behavior, and mental ability. Wouldn't you like to see your children pulling higher grades in school? This is exactly what happened in Wisconsin when a local bread baker started including flaxseed in his bakery products and donating them to local elementary schools. The parents and teachers also noted that the children's attendance and behavior had improved.

Research done by a prominent psychologist found that the essential fats improved the psychological conditions of his mentally challenged patients. Athletes have noticed improved performance and decreased muscle fatigue as a result of the fats in flax improving the availability of oxygen to their hard-working muscles. Patients with the deadly disease lupus nephritis have reason for optimism after research showed that flax oil could decrease mortality caused by their disease by over 60 percent!

What about relief from inflammation and arthritis pain? Flax delicately balances hormones in the body that aggravate these conditions. Persons suffering from skin conditions, such as psoriasis and eczema, have also found relief with flax oil supplementation.

I could continue on and on extolling the benefits of flax. The essential good fats have been found to be therapeutic in over 60 diseases and illnesses. The main point I would like you to remember is that you can avoid the majority of these health challenges by following a healthful diet with the inclusion of flax oil. This section is designed to serve as a tool to help you incorporate the highly important essential fatty acids in the form of flax oil into everyday wholesome foods.

Flax oil is quickly becoming one of the most popular health foods in our country. Research scientists continue to learn of its practically unlimited potential in human nutrition. Many leading health and nutrition authorities are recommending flax oil as an integral part of a foundation for a healthy diet. The excitement triggered by flax is truly causing a "fat revolution" away from no fat and low fat to the right fat, as found most abundantly in flax.

The growing popularity of flax has not gone unnoticed by food manufacturers wanting to boost the nutritional value of the foods they offer to consumers. While flax does not lend itself to modern manufacturing and refinement, flaxseed has been used successfully in baked goods, and flax oil seems a perfect ingredient for salad dressings. Health-conscious companies are working to make the consumption of flaxseed and flax oil more practical to consumers. It would appear that our 100-year departure from the essential fats has come full circle. The bottom line is that flax is here to stay, and you can expect to hear more about its amazing attributes.

I imagine you are all thinking, "This sounds too good to be true—flax oil sure sounds like a panacea."

Flax oil, along with the essential fatty acids it contains, is just one more example of the truly unbelievable healing power of natural, unrefined foods. In fact, if our food wasn't so heavily refined, we wouldn't be faced with the illnesses that the essential fatty acids and other valuable nutrients so powerfully protect us against.

We also must remember that the essential fatty acids found in flax oil are truly essential to life, and we must get them in our foods in order to appreciate optimal, vibrant health and long life. Is it important to reintroduce these nutrient powerhouses, the essential fatty acids, back into our diet? You bet it is, and you can start right here and right now!

Consider the impact you can have on your health and the health of your loved ones by simply committing to get as little as one tablespoon of unrefined flax oil in your daily diet. What a small price to pay for protection against cancer, heart disease, stroke, and other devastating illnesses. Thousands of folks across the country have been experiencing the profound health effects associated with this remarkable food—not to mention the beautifying effects it can have.

In *The Healing Power of Flax* you are presented with simple and practical ways to incorporate flax oil into your daily diet. You will learn how to easily add this healing and protective food with fun, easy-to-prepare, and delicious snacks, dips, soups, and meals. You can find unrefined, organic, expeller pressed flax oil at most health food stores, usually located in the refrigerator section.

I know you will agree with me that we have been deprived of our essential fatty acids for too long. It's high time to put the fat back, the right fat that is, as found in unrefined flax oil.

Long and vibrant health to you and yours.

*Bon appétit!*

# CHAPTER TWENTY-TWO

# Breakfast and Breads

*Start your day supercharged with the right fat found in flax*

## BREAKFAST AND BREADS RECIPE INDEX

## FLAX FOR THOUGHT

Breakfast is considered by many health experts to be the most important meal of the day. We are literally breaking an approximately 12-hour fast from the day before. Breakfast serves to raise, and hopefully sustain, our blood sugar and energy levels until the noon hour. The addition of flaxseed and flax oil to breakfast foods serves several important functions.

- The essential fats in flax are able to help you maintain consistent energy and blood sugar levels throughout the day.
- The addition of flax to children's diets has been discovered to improve learning ability and behavior. What a great head start to your child's school day!
- The ingestion of foods with flax oil causes a feeling of fullness and fulfillment that follows a satisfying meal.
- The essential fatty acids in flax help to decrease the "stickiness" of blood platelets. The morning hours are considered the most dangerous for risk of heart attack because of sluggish blood flow caused by sticky blood platelets.

Breakfast lends itself well to the addition of flax oil. Here are a few quick and easy ways to improvise with flax at breakfast time.

- Combine one part chilled flax oil with one part melted butter, then chill. The new spread will resemble the consistency of margarine—without all the toxic funny fats and with the addition of the vital essential fatty acids. Use this spread on toast, on baked potatoes, or for any other low-heat application where you would ordinarily use butter or margarine.
- Combine one part flax oil with one part pure maple syrup. You will now have a buttery-tasting maple syrup topping for waffles, French toast, and pancakes. It's a terrific way to sneak the essential fatty acids into your child's diet.
- For a quick, easy, and healthy breakfast, simply stir one tablespoon of flax oil into yogurt and top with your favorite fruit.
- Mix flax oil with your favorite hot cereal for a buttery consistency and nutty flavor.
- For recipes that call for ground flaxseed, simply place whole flaxseed in a coffee grinder and grind until desired consistency is achieved.

### Granola-Like Breakfast

| | |
|---|---|
| 4 tablespoons sesame seeds | 1/4 cup fresh apple juice |
| 4 tablespoons sunflower seeds | cinnamon to taste |
| 4 tablespoons flaxseed | 1 cup fresh fruit |
| 4 cups rolled oats | plain nonfat yogurt to top |

- Grind the sesame seeds, sunflower seeds, and flaxseed in a coffee grinder.
- Combine the seed mixture with the oats. Divide into 2 equal portions.
- Soak one portion with the apple juice.
- Place both portions in the refrigerator overnight.
- Stir the portions together. Add the cinnamon and fresh fruit.
- Top with yogurt.

*SERVES 4*

## Fresh Fruit Breakfast Muesli

*Flax meal muesli*

> 2 tablespoons flaxseed
>
> 1 tablespoon raw honey

- Grind the flaxseed to a coarse consistency in a coffee grinder.
- Place in a serving dish. Add the honey. Combine by thoroughly mashing with a fork.

*Yogurt filling*

> 4 ounces plain or vanilla nonfat yogurt
>
> 3 tablespoons Barlean's organic flax oil
>
> 1 teaspoon raw honey

- Combine all ingredients in a small mixing bowl. Whisk or hand blend to an even consistency.
- Pour over the flax meal muesli.

*Toppings*

| | | | |
|---|---|---|---|
| banana slices | cherries | peach slices | peanuts |
| blackberries | currants | pear slices | pecans |
| blueberries | fruit juice | cinnamon | pine nuts |
| raspberries | grapes | ginger | slivered almonds |
| strawberries | grated apple | nutmeg | walnuts |

- Top the muesli with the toppings of your choice.

*SERVES 2*

## Banana, Apple, and Date Breakfast Pudding

*A breakfast or anytime treat, tasty and chewy.*

> 3 large dates, pits removed
>
> 1 apple, diced
>
> 1 large frozen banana
>
> 3 sections of an orange
>
> 1 1/2 tablespoons Barlean's organic flax oil
>
> yogurt and walnuts to top (optional)

- Place all ingredients in a blender or food processor and process to desired consistency.
- Serve in a bowl or a tall glass.
- Top with yogurt and walnuts if desired.

*SERVES 1 TO 2*

## Apple Muesli

*Popularized in Europe, muesli is a tremendously healthy way to start your day.*

2 tablespoons oatmeal

4 teaspoons water

2 apples

2 1/2 tablespoons wheat germ

juice of 1/2 lemon

3/4 cup yogurt

1 tablespoon raisins

2 tablespoons Barlean's organic flax oil

2 tablespoons raw honey

3 tablespoons chopped walnuts

- Soak the oatmeal overnight in the water.
- Grate the apple or process in a food processor.
- Combine all ingredients and mix well. Eat immediately.

*SERVES 2*

## Fruit Lupes

*A delicious fruit cereal the way Mother Nature intended.*

2 large crisp apples, cored

1 tablespoon currants

1/4 cup shredded coconut

1/4 cup diced dried figs

1/4 cup coarsely ground almonds

1/2 teaspoon cinnamon

1/4 cup apple juice

2 teaspoons pure maple syrup

2 teaspoons Barlean's organic flax oil

- Place the apples and currants in a food processor and coarsely grind.
- Combine the apple mixture with the coconut, figs, almonds, cinnamon, and apple juice.
- In a small bowl or cup, thoroughly blend the maple syrup and flax oil.
- Add the flax-maple syrup mixture to the other ingredients. Mix well and serve.

*SERVES 2*

## Hot Carob Cereal

*A rich and warming cereal.*

2 1/4 cups water or rice milk

1 cup oatmeal

1 tablespoon unsweetened carob powder

1/2 teaspoon cinnamon

2 tablespoons Barlean's organic flax oil

1 tablespoon raisins

2 teaspoons raw honey

plain nonfat yogurt to top (optional)

- Bring the water or rice milk to a boil. Stir in the oatmeal, carob powder, and cinnamon. Cook for 3 minutes.
- Remove from heat and stir in the flax oil, raisins, and honey. Let sit with lid on for 1 minute.
- Serve topped with yogurt if desired.

*SERVES 2*

## Happy Apple Breakfast

*Other rolled grains such as wheat, barley, rye, or triticale can be used in various combinations instead of some or all of the rolled oats. All of these grains have the same cooking characteristics.*

1¹/₂ cups rolled oats

2¹/₂ cups water, milk, or apple juice

1 medium green or golden apple, sliced

¹/₄ cup currants, raisins, or chopped dates

¹/₄ cup freshly roasted pumpkin seeds (optional)

2 tablespoons Barlean's organic flax oil

raw honey to sweeten

plain nonfat yogurt to top (optional)

- Combine all ingredients, except the flax oil and honey, in a saucepan. Simmer on the stove for 10 minutes. Cover and let sit for 5 minutes.
- Stir in the flax oil and honey to taste.
- Serve topped with yogurt if desired.

*SERVES 2*

## Buttery Banana Pancakes

*The illusion of buttery-rich pancakes made easy by combining maple syrup with flax oil.*

### Syrup

¹/₄ cup pure maple syrup

¹/₄ cup Barlean's organic flax oil

### Pancakes

1¹/₂ cups whole wheat pastry flour

¹/₄ teaspoon salt or salt substitute

3 teaspoons baking powder

1³/₄ cups rice milk, soy milk, or nonfat milk

1 tablespoon butter or extra virgin olive oil

1¹/₂ ripe bananas, sliced

- Whisk the maple syrup together with the flax oil until thoroughly blended.
- Combine the flour, salt, and baking powder. Sift into a mixing bowl.
- Pour the milk into the flour mixture and mix until thoroughly combined.
- Lightly butter or oil a griddle and preheat to medium heat.
- Pour ¹/₄ cup of the batter at a time onto the griddle. Add the banana slices randomly to the top of the pancake. Cook about 3 minutes until the bottom is lightly browned. Turn over and cook until the second side is lightly browned.
- Serve at once. Top liberally with flax-maple syrup.

*SERVES 2 TO 3*

---

### Barlean Butter

*At last, a spreadable alternative to margarine with half the saturated fat of butter. Use on toast, bagels, or muffins.*

1 stick of butter

4 ounces Barlean's organic flax oil

- Cut the butter into cubes and gently melt in a small saucepan.
- Pour the liquefied butter into a small, sealable container.
- Stir in the flax oil. Seal and set in the refrigerator to solidify.

---

### French Toast with Flax-Maple Syrup

*French toast with a buttery-like maple syrup made by adding flax oil.*

**Syrup**

1/4 cup pure maple syrup

1/4 cup Barlean's organic flax oil

**French toast**

1/2 cup whole wheat pastry flour

1/4 teaspoon salt or salt substitute

1 cup rice milk or soy milk

6 slices whole-grain bread

cinnamon and nutmeg to taste

- Whisk the maple syrup together with the flax oil until thoroughly blended.
- Mix the flour and salt in a bowl large enough to accommodate one piece of toast. Aerate the mixture with a wire whisk.
- Pour the milk into the center of the flour and mix briskly.
- Let the batter sit for 20 minutes.
- Heat a lightly buttered griddle. Mix the batter well. Dip each slice of bread in batter to coat completely. Cook about 3 minutes until the first side is lightly browned, then turn over and cook the second side.
- Sprinkle with cinnamon and nutmeg to taste.
- Top French toast with flax-maple syrup.

*SERVES 2 TO 3*

## Vanilla-Raisin Cream of Rice

*A hot and healthy rice cereal.*

| | |
|---|---|
| 1 cup organic brown rice | 2 teaspoons vanilla extract |
| 3¹/₂ cups water, soy milk, rice milk, or milk | 4 tablespoons Barlean's organic flax oil |
| ¹/₂ cup raisins | plain nonfat yogurt to top |

- Finely grind the rice to a powdery consistency in a blender, coffee grinder, or nut/seed grinder.
- Bring the water or milk to a boil in a large pot. Whisk in the rice powder. Add the raisins. Cover and simmer for 15 minutes.
- Remove from heat. Stir in the vanilla and flax oil.
- Serve immediately.
- Top with yogurt to complete the oil/protein combination.

*SERVES 3 TO 4*

## Barlean's Best Oatmeal

*A delicious, nutty-flavored hot breakfast cereal. An incredibly healthy way to start a new day.*

| | |
|---|---|
| 1 cup oat groats (whole oat grain) | dash of cinnamon |
| 4 cups rice milk, soy milk, milk, or water | raw honey to flavor |
| ¹/₂ cup raisins | 4 tablespoons Barlean's organic flax oil |
| ¹/₂ teaspoon vanilla | plain nonfat yogurt to top |

- Grind the oat groats in a blender or coffee grinder to desired consistency (depending on your preference for coarse or fine cereal).
- Bring the milk or water to a rolling boil. Whisk the ground oats into the milk. Add the raisins. Reduce heat and simmer for 20 minutes.
- Remove from heat. Add the vanilla, cinnamon, and honey. Stir in the flax oil.
- Serve topped with yogurt.

*SERVES 4*

---

## Barlean's Quick and Easy Oatmeal

*A quick and simple version of Barlean's Best Oatmeal.*

| | |
|---|---|
| 1 cup quick oats | dash of cinnamon |
| 2 cups rice milk, soy milk, milk, or water | raw honey to flavor |
| 1/4 cup raisins | 2 tablespoons Barlean's organic flax oil |
| 1/4 teaspoon vanilla | plain nonfat yogurt to top |

- Combine the oats, milk, and raisins in a saucepan.
- Bring to a boil. Cook about 1 minute over medium heat, stirring occasionally.
- Remove from heat. Add the vanilla, cinnamon, and honey. Stir in the flax oil.
- Serve topped with yogurt.

*SERVES 2 TO 3*

---

## Quick Bread

| | |
|---|---|
| 2 cups ground flaxseed* | grated peel from 2 lemons (save lemons for juice) |
| 1 cup whole wheat flour | 1/2 cup raw honey or sugar |
| 1 cup all-purpose flour | 2 cups raisins, chopped prunes or dates |
| 1 teaspoon salt | (soak ahead a few minutes; drain) |
| 2 teaspoons baking soda | express lemons for juice, adding enough |
| 4 egg whites or 2 eggs | buttermilk to yield 1 1/2 cups liquid |

* *Grind whole flaxseed to the consistency of flour in a coffee grinder.*
- Combine ingredients in descending order and mix thoroughly.
- Bake in 6 lightly buttered, small loaf pans (approximately 3" x 7") for 40 minutes at 325°F.

*MAKES 6 SMALL LOAVES*

## Wheat-Free Flax Bread

*A recipe for people on a wheat-free diet.*

1/2 cup beaten mashed potatoes
   (or 2 tablespoons dry instant mashed potatoes)
1/4 cup butter
1/4 cup sugar
1/2 cup cooked white rice
6 eggs, separated
1 1/2 cups brown rice flour
2 tablespoons soy flour

3 teaspoons baking powder
1 teaspoon baking soda
1 teaspoon cream of tartar
1/2 teaspoon salt
1/8 teaspoon black pepper (optional)
3/4 cup milk (if using instant potatoes
   add another 1/2 cup milk)
1/4 cup flaxseed

- If using instant mashed potatoes, reconstitute with the additional 1/2 cup milk.
- Be sure that the potatoes are free of lumps. Cream the potatoes thoroughly with the butter and sugar. Mix in the white rice, then add the egg yolks one at a time, beating thoroughly after each one.
- Sift the dry ingredients together and add to the potato mixture alternately with the milk.
- Beat the egg whites to hold their shape in soft (not stiff) peaks. Fold in the egg whites. Fold in the flaxseed. Pour the batter into 2 lightly buttered 9 1/2" x 5" loaf pans. Bake at 350°F for about 1 hour.

*MAKES 2 LOAVES*

## Whole-Grain Flax Bread

1 1/4 cups ground flaxseed*
5 cups warm water
4 tablespoons softened raw honey
2 1/2 tablespoons instant yeast
1 cup oatmeal

4 cups unbleached white flour
1/2 cup whey powder
2 teaspoons salt
8 cups stone-ground whole wheat
   flour (approximately)

- * Grind whole flaxseed to a fine consistency in a coffee grinder.
- Combine the water, honey, and yeast. Let sit for 3 to 4 minutes.
- In a separate bowl, mix the oatmeal, unbleached flour, ground flaxseed, whey powder, and salt. Add these dry ingredients to the yeast mixture and mix well.
- Beat for 5 minutes by hand, then add the whole wheat flour and mix until dough is quite stiff. (If using a bread kneading machine, add the whole wheat flour and mix on high speed for 5 minutes.) Knead. Let rise 15 minutes. Punch down and let rise another 15 minutes. Punch down and shape into loaves.
- Let the bread rise until doubled in size. Bake loaves at 350°F for 40 to 45 minutes.

*MAKES 2 LOAVES*

### Flax Bagels

½ cup ground flaxseed*

2¼ cups flour

1 teaspoon salt

1 package yeast

2¼ cups water (110°F to 130°F)

additional flour for kneading

¼ cup sugar

* *Grind whole flaxseed to the consistency of flour in a coffee grinder.*

- Using an electric mixer on low speed for 1 minute, mix the flour, ground flaxseed, salt, yeast, and water. Scrape the bowl, then mix on high speed for 2 to 3 minutes. Add additional flour as needed.
- Place the dough on a floured surface. Knead, adding flour as necessary to form a stiff dough that is smooth and pliable. Place in a greased bowl and cover with a damp, warm towel. Let sit in a warm spot for 10 minutes.
- Working quickly, divide the dough into 12 pieces. Roll each into a ball and punch a hole in the center of the ball with a floured finger.
- Pull the dough gently to form a 2-inch circle. Place on a greased baking sheet. Let rise for 30 to 45 minutes.
- While the dough is rising, bring 6 cups of water to a boil in a large skillet or Dutch oven. Add the sugar. Reduce heat so the water is at a simmer.
- After the bagels have risen, place in the simmering water for 5 minutes, turning once. Remove and place on a wire rack for 3 to 5 minutes.
- Place on a baking sheet and bake in a preheated oven at 375°F for 25 to 30 minutes. When done the bagels should be a golden color.
- If desired, garlic, onion, sesame seeds, herbs, spices, or other flavors may be added to the dry ingredients. Use approximately 1 to 1½ teaspoons of flavor. Sprinkle seeds on bagels after boiling and prior to baking if a topping is desired.

*MAKES 12 BAGELS*

———~———

## Flax and Potato Bread

1/4 cup flaxseed

3/4 cup water

1 1/2 cups flour

hot water (approximately 130°F)

2 tablespoons potato flakes

3 tablespoons raw honey

1 tablespoon nonfat milk powder

1 package instant yeast

1 teaspoon salt

1 teaspoon butter

additional flour for kneading

- In a large mixing bowl, soak the flaxseed in warm water for 45 minutes, then add the remaining ingredients.
- Mix with an electric mixer for 1/2 minute. Scrape the bowl and mix on high speed for another 2 to 3 minutes.
- While mixing with a spoon, add additional flour to make a dough you can work by hand.
- Place the dough on a floured surface and knead by hand. Add additional flour to make a stiff, pliable dough.
- Place the dough in a greased bowl. Cover and set aside in a warm spot for 20 minutes.
- Divide the dough into 2 equal pieces. Place in lightly buttered 4 1/4" x 8 1/4" bread pans.
- Set in a warm place with no cool draft until doubled in size.
- Bake at 380°F for 25 minutes or until the crust is a golden color.

*MAKES 2 LOAVES*

———~———

## Multigrain Bread

1/2 cup ground flaxseed*

2 cups whole wheat flour

1/2 cup rye flour

1/2 cup oat bran (optional)

4 1/2 cups high-gluten bread flour

1/4 cup sugar

1/4 cup molasses

1/4 cup unrefined canola oil

1 tablespoon dry yeast

2 1/4 cups warm water

* *Grind whole flaxseed to the consistency of fine flour in a coffee grinder.*

- Combine ingredients in descending order and mix thoroughly.
- Pour dough into 3 standard-size, lightly buttered bread pans.
- Bake at 375°F for about 1 hour or until loaves are loose in pans.

MAKES 3 LOAVES

CHAPTER TWENTY-THREE

# Dips and Dressings

## A quick, easy, and practical way
## to get your daily dose of essential fatty acids

### DIPS AND DRESSINGS RECIPE INDEX

### FLAX FOR THOUGHT

Dips and salad dressings can harbor many hidden sources of unnatural and dangerous fats and oils in our diet. But, on the other hand, they can become some of our strongest allies in bringing the right fats, the essential fatty acids, back into our diets if they are made with flax oil. Until dips and salad dressings are made available with unrefined flax and vegetable oils, we should fashion our own blends with the recipes found in this chapter.

Here are a couple of tips regarding dips and dressings.

- To ensure healthful salad dressings when dining out, take along your homemade blend in a tightly sealed plastic container.
- After making your dips and salad dressings from healthful oils, be sure to refrigerate them to extend shelf life.

### Flax-Almond Mayonnaise

*A rich, creamy, and tasty alternative to mayonnaise made with processed oils. Use whenever mayonnaise is called for.*

1/4 cup raw almonds

1/4 cup water, soy milk, or rice milk

1/2 teaspoon nutritional yeast

1/4 teaspoon garlic powder

1/4 teaspoon salt or salt substitute

1/4 cup Barlean's organic flax oil

1/4 cup extra virgin olive oil

2 tablespoons lemon juice

1/4 teaspoon apple cider vinegar

- Combine ingredients in a blender or food processor in descending order. Blend on high speed until thick and creamy.
- Refrigerate until ready to use. Keeps 10 days to 2 weeks refrigerated.

*MAKES 1 CUP*

### Fresh Mexican Salsa

*A zesty traditional Mexican salsa made even better with the addition of flax oil. Great as a dip for tortilla chips or as a sauce on enchiladas, burritos, and tacos.*

3 tomatoes, diced

4 sprigs fresh cilantro

1/2 medium onion, diced

1 scallion, chopped

1 small jalapeño pepper

1/2 cup tomato sauce

3 tablespoons Barlean's organic flax oil

- Combine the tomatoes, cilantro, onion, scallion, and jalapeño pepper in a blender or food processor and process to desired consistency, chunky or saucy.
- In a separate bowl, combine the tomato sauce and flax oil. Stir to a uniform consistency.
- Mix everything together and chill until ready to serve.

*MAKES 2 CUPS*

---

### Bean Dip

*Serve this dip with tortilla chips or firm vegetables, such as celery, carrots, and bell peppers.*

1 16-ounce can or 2 cups cooked cannellini beans (white kidney beans), drained and rinsed

4 large cloves garlic, boiled for 5 minutes, then peeled and sliced

2 tablespoons Barlean's organic flax oil

1/4 to 1/2 teaspoon hot pepper sauce

1 to 2 teaspoons minced jalapeño pepper (fresh or canned)

- Combine all ingredients in a food processor and blend until smooth.

*MAKES ABOUT 2 CUPS*

---

### Hummus

*A fantastic-tasting Middle Eastern dish to be used as a dip or as a filling in pita sandwiches. An excellent source of complete protein and, now, essential fatty acids.*

1 15-ounce can or 1 2/3 cups cooked garbanzo beans (chickpeas)

1/4 cup tahini (sesame seed paste)

3 tablespoons lemon juice

3 tablespoons Barlean's organic flax oil

2 medium cloves garlic

1/4 teaspoon ground coriander

1/4 teaspoon ground cumin

1/4 teaspoon paprika

dash of cayenne

1/4 cup minced scallions

2 tablespoons minced fresh parsley for garnish

- In a blender or food processor, process the garbanzo beans, tahini, lemon juice, and flax oil until the mixture reaches the consistency of a coarse paste. Use as much of the garbanzo liquid, or water, as needed.
- Add the garlic, coriander, cumin, paprika, and cayenne and blend thoroughly.
- Transfer the hummus to a bowl and stir in the scallions.
- Cover the hummus and refrigerate.
- Garnish with parsley before serving.

*MAKES ABOUT 2 1/2 CUPS*

## Dairyless Flax Sour Cream

*An alternative for those sensitive to dairy products or those wanting to avoid animal products. All the tang you'd expect from sour cream.*

6 ounces silken tofu

1 tablespoon Barlean's organic flax oil

1 tablespoon nutritional yeast

2 tablespoons lemon juice

2 teaspoons rice vinegar

1 teaspoon plum vinegar

salt or salt substitute to taste

chives for garnish (optional)

- Steam the tofu for 2 minutes.
- Combine all ingredients in a blender or food processor and process on high speed for 1 minute.
- Garnish each serving with chives if desired.

*MAKES 1 CUP*

## Dairyless Sour Cream and Onion Dip

*A dairyless alternative to sour cream.*

1/2 cup Dairyless Flax Sour Cream (above)

1 small clove garlic, pressed

1/2 cup minced scallions

1/2 cup Flax-Almond Mayonnaise (page 137)

1 teaspoon Worcestershire sauce

- Combine all ingredients in a blender or food processor and process until thick and creamy. Flavor is enhanced if allowed to sit awhile before serving.
- Keeps 1 to 2 days refrigerated.

*MAKES 1 1/2 CUPS*

## Almond-Flax Butter

*Produces a wonderful balance of omega-3, 6, and 9 fatty acids. Extraordinary spread over toasted bread, as a vegetable dip, or used in place of peanut butter.*

1/2 cup raw almonds

3 tablespoons Barlean's organic flax oil

- Grind the almonds to the consistency of meal in a blender or food processor. Add the flax oil and process until creamy.

## Middle Eastern Bean Dip

*Rich in protein and essential fatty acids. Good as an appetizer before a salad or vegetable meal. Use as a sand-wich filling, cracker spread, or dip for chips.*

1 cup dried fava beans or whole lentils

2 tablespoons Barlean's organic flax oil

1 tablespoon lemon juice

1 clove garlic, crushed

1 tablespoon finely chopped fresh parsley

1 teaspoon raw honey

salt or salt substitute to taste

freshly ground black pepper to taste

4 pitted ripe olives for garnish

- Cover the beans generously with boiling water and leave them to soak 4 to 5 hours if possible. (Not as long if you are using lentils.) Drain and rinse.
- Place the beans or lentils in a medium saucepan with plenty of water and simmer over gentle heat until tender. (About 1¼ to 1½ hours for beans, 30 to 45 minutes for lentils.) Drain, reserving the liquid.
- In a bowl, combine the beans or lentils with the flax oil, lemon juice, garlic, parsley, honey, salt, and pepper. Mash and mix thoroughly and, if necessary, add enough of the reserved cooking liquid to make a thick, creamy paste.
- Smooth the surface of the mixture and garnish with olives.

*MAKES ABOUT 1½ CUPS*

## Green Pea Guacamole

*Can be used as an inexpensive substitute to traditional avocado guacamole. Contains healthful essential fatty acids.*

1 cup green peas (fresh or frozen)

¼ cup water (from steaming the peas)

1 jalapeño pepper, seeds removed

½ tablespoon lemon juice

1 tablespoon (packed) chopped
   fresh cilantro leaves

2 to 3 tablespoons chopped onion

2 tablespoons Barlean's organic flax oil

dash of cumin powder

dash of salt or salt substitute

2 cloves garlic, pressed

cilantro, cayenne, and a wedge of lime for garnish

- In a small pan of water, steam the peas for 3 minutes until tender. Drain, reserving ¼ cup of the steaming water.
- Place the peas and the ¼ cup of the steaming water in a food processor and puree. Add the remain-ing ingredients and puree to a thick, even consistency.
- Transfer to a small bowl and garnish with cilantro, cayenne, and a lime wedge.

*SERVES 3*

## Eggplant Dip

*Wonderful as a vegetable dip or sandwich spread.*

1 eggplant

2 medium cloves garlic, crushed

1 scallion, chopped

1/4 cup chopped fresh parsley

1 tablespoon lemon juice

3 tablespoons Barlean's organic flax oil

1/2 teaspoon dried dill weed

- Bake eggplant at 400°F for 1 hour or until soft.
- Remove from oven and when cool enough to handle, peel and dice.
- Place all ingredients in a blender or food processor and process until smooth.
- Chill and serve.

*MAKES ABOUT 2 CUPS*

## Eggplant and Tahini Cream

*The subtle flavor of eggplant blends wonderfully with the rich, earthy taste of tahini. This dish is perfect with warm pita bread or crisp toast and makes a good light lunch served with soup.*

2 medium eggplants (about 1 pound)

2 heaping tablespoons tahini

2 tablespoons Barlean's organic flax oil

1 tablespoon lemon juice

1 large clove garlic, crushed

salt or salt substitute to taste

freshly ground black pepper to taste

lettuce leaves

sesame seeds (optional)

fresh parsley and chives for garnish

- Prick the eggplants and bake at 400°F for 30 minutes. Let them cool, then remove the skins.
- Combine the eggplant, tahini, flax oil, lemon juice, and garlic in a blender or food processor and process until smooth.
- Season the mixture with salt and pepper to taste, then chill.
- When ready to serve, arrange a bed of lettuce leaves on a small plate and spoon the mixture on top. Sprinkle with sesame seeds and garnish with parsley and chives.

*MAKES ABOUT 2 1/2 CUPS*

## Spicy Pinto Bean Dip

*Serve with no-oil tortilla chips.*

2½ cups cooked pinto beans, drained

1½ tablespoons crushed garlic

2 teaspoons onion powder

3 tablespoons Barlean's organic flax oil

1½ teaspoons ground cumin

2 teaspoons diced jalapeño pepper

1 teaspoon salt or salt substitute

¼ cup water

3 tablespoons brown rice vinegar

dash of chili powder

cayenne or paprika for garnish

- Combine all ingredients in a blender or food processor and puree until smooth.
- Transfer to a bowl and garnish with cayenne or paprika.

*MAKES ABOUT 3 CUPS*

## Thai Tomato Salsa

*Serve over steamed vegetables and rice, broiled or roasted chicken, or fish.*

2 scallions (3 inches of green left on), slivered lengthwise

⅓ cup lemon juice

3 tomatoes, diced

1 to 2 bunches fresh cilantro leaves, minced

3 to 4 cloves garlic, crushed

6 large basil leaves, finely chopped

⅓ large red onion, diced

1 tablespoon peeled and grated fresh ginger

1 tablespoon balsamic vinegar

¼ cup Barlean's organic flax oil

¼ cup extra virgin olive oil

salt or salt substitute to taste

freshly ground black pepper to taste

- Soak the scallions in the lemon juice for 30 minutes. Drain, reserving half of the lemon juice.
- Mince the scallions.
- In a medium bowl, combine the scallions, reserved lemon juice, and the remaining ingredients.

*MAKES ABOUT 2 CUPS*

## Spinach-Mushroom Dip

*Can be served as an appetizer on crackers, as a filling for sandwiches, or as a dip for chips.*

1 clove garlic, crushed

1 cup chopped onion

1/2 pound mushrooms, cleaned and chopped

1 tablespoon butter

1 1/4 cups spinach (or 10 ounces frozen)

1/4 cup broth or white wine

1 cup water

1/2 cup tahini

1 teaspoon salt or salt substitute

1/4 cup nutritional yeast flakes

4 tablespoons Barlean's organic flax oil

3 tablespoons lemon juice

1/8 teaspoon cayenne

1/2 teaspoon dried dill weed

- Sauté the garlic, onion, and mushrooms in the butter over low heat until soft.
- Steam the spinach until wilted.
- Combine all ingredients in a blender or food processor and puree until creamy.
- Chill and serve.

*MAKES ABOUT 4 CUPS*

## Sunflower Seed Dressing

1 cup hulled sunflower seeds

1/2 cup Barlean's organic flax oil

1/4 cup lemon juice

1/2 cup soft tofu

1 tablespoon soy sauce or tamari

1/2 tablespoon water

1/2 teaspoon dried basil

1/2 teaspoon dried thyme

- Combine all ingredients in a blender or food processor and process until creamy.

*MAKES ABOUT 2 CUPS*

## Basil Dressing

1/4 cup Barlean's organic flax oil

1/4 cup water

3 tablespoons lemon juice

2 tablespoons fresh basil or 2 teaspoons dried basil

1 teaspoon finely chopped garlic

freshly ground black pepper to taste

- Combine all ingredients in a blender or food processor and blend thoroughly.

*MAKES ABOUT 3/4 CUP*

## Lemon-Tarragon Dressing

1/4 cup lemon juice

2 tablespoons water

1 teaspoon Dijon mustard

cayenne to taste

2 tablespoons Barlean's organic flax oil

1 1/2 teaspoons chopped fresh tarragon

or 1/2 teaspoon dried tarragon

- Combine the lemon juice, water, mustard, and cayenne in a blender and blend thoroughly. Add the flax oil and tarragon and blend well.

*MAKES 1/2 CUP*

## Green Goddess Taiwanese Style

*Try over salads or as a dip for Thai spring rolls.*

1 1/2 tablespoons peanut butter

1 tablespoon golden miso

1 teaspoon peeled and chopped fresh ginger

3/4 cup water

1 tablespoon rice vinegar

2 tablespoons Barlean's organic flax oil

1/4 teaspoon red chili flakes

1/2 cup chopped scallions

1 teaspoon raw honey

3 tablespoons lime juice

- Combine all ingredients in a blender or food processor and process until creamy.

*MAKES ABOUT 1 3/4 CUPS*

## Oregano Dressing

3 tablespoons red wine vinegar or rice vinegar

1 tablespoon water

1 tablespoon lemon juice

3 tablespoons Barlean's organic flax oil

2 tablespoons minced fresh parsley

1 tablespoon chopped fresh oregano

or 3/4 teaspoon dried oregano

freshly ground black pepper to taste

- Combine all ingredients in a blender and blend thoroughly.

*MAKES 3/4 CUP*

## Miso-Ginger Dressing

1 cup water

1 1/2 tablespoons mellow white miso

1 tablespoon tahini

2 cloves garlic, chopped

1/2 tablespoon peeled and chopped fresh ginger

1 tablespoon lemon juice

1/2 scallion, chopped

3 tablespoons Barlean's organic flax oil

- Combine all ingredients in a blender or food processor and process until creamy.

*MAKES 1 1/3 CUPS*

### Cucumber-Dill Dressing

2 tablespoons lemon juice

3 tablespoons Barlean's organic flax oil

2 tablespoons extra virgin olive oil

1 medium cucumber, peeled and diced

1 tablespoon mayonnaise or eggless mayonnaise

1/4 teaspoon dry mustard

2 teaspoons dried dill weed
    or 2 tablespoons fresh dill

1/4 teaspoon salt or salt substitute

- Combine all ingredients in a blender or food processor and process to a creamy consistency.

*MAKES ABOUT 1 CUP*

### Herbal Bouquet Salad Dressing

2 cloves garlic, crushed

1/4 cup Barlean's organic flax oil

1/4 cup extra virgin olive oil

4 tablespoons lemon juice

1/2 teaspoon dried basil

1/2 teaspoon dried chervil

1/4 teaspoon dried thyme

1/4 teaspoon dried oregano

1/2 teaspoon dried savory

1/4 teaspoon ground coriander

1/8 teaspoon dried sage

salt or salt substitute to taste

2 teaspoons Dijon mustard

1 tablespoon mayonnaise or eggless mayonnaise

- Combine all ingredients in a blender or food processor and process to an even consistency.

*MAKES ABOUT 3/4 CUP*

### Creamy Garlic Dressing

*A dairyless salad dressing that mimics the richness and texture of sour cream.*

1/4 cup water

1 medium clove garlic, crushed

4 ounces soft tofu or silken tofu

1/4 cup Barlean's organic flax oil

3 tablespoons lemon juice

2 teaspoons rice vinegar

1 teaspoon kelp

1 tablespoon poppy seeds

1 teaspoon dried dill weed

seasoned salt or salt substitute to taste (optional)

- Combine all ingredients in a blender or food processor and process to an even consistency.

*MAKES 1 1/2 CUPS*

## Lemon–Poppy Seed Dressing

1½ tablespoons poppy seeds

2½ tablespoons lemon juice

1 teaspoon raw honey

2 tablespoons mayonnaise or eggless mayonnaise

½ teaspoon dry mustard

1½ tablespoons Barlean's organic flax oil

• Combine all ingredients and whisk vigorously.

*MAKES ABOUT ³/4 CUP*

## Tomato Salad Dressing

½ cup tomato juice

¼ cup Barlean's organic flax oil

¼ cup extra virgin olive oil

3 tablespoons lemon juice

½ teaspoon dried basil

¼ teaspoon dried oregano

1 clove garlic, crushed

• Combine all ingredients in a blender or food processor and blend for 2 minutes.

*MAKES ABOUT 1 CUP*

## Cilantro Dressing

*Flavorful with accents of the southwest.*

3 tablespoons tahini

1½ tablespoons miso

1 large clove garlic

¾ cup water

¼ cup rice vinegar

⅓ cup (packed) fresh cilantro leaves

dash of hot chili sauce

2 tablespoons Barlean's organic flax oil

• Combine all ingredients in a blender or food processor and process until creamy.

*MAKES 1¹/3 CUPS*

## Dreamy Creamy Avocado Dressing

1 large ripe avocado, diced

1 medium cucumber, peeled and cut in chunks

2 teaspoons dried dill weed

seasoned salt or salt-free seasoning to taste

1 tablespoon lime juice

2 tablespoons Barlean's organic flax oil

• Combine all ingredients in a blender or food processor and process to a smooth, even consistency.

*MAKES ABOUT 1¹/2 CUPS*

## Herb Oil

*Serve on fish, potatoes, and vegetables. Expensive Italian restaurants serve warm herbed oil to dip bread into. Try it, it's a real treat!*

<sup></sup>

| | |
|---|---|
| 1/2 teaspoon dried savory | 1 tablespoon minced chives |
| 1/2 teaspoon dried marjoram | 1 clove garlic, crushed |
| 1/2 teaspoon dried basil | 1/4 teaspoon paprika |
| 1/2 teaspoon dried tarragon | 1/4 cup Barlean's organic flax oil |
| 1 tablespoon minced fresh parsley | |

- Pulverize the dried herbs by rubbing between palms of hands.
- Combine all ingredients. Store in a covered jar and keep in the refrigerator.

*MAKES ABOUT 1/4 CUP*

*Contributed by Dr. Jack Tips, N.D., The Pro Vita Plan*

## Orange–Sesame Seed Dressing

3/4 cup orange juice (about 2 oranges juiced)

1/4 cup Barlean's organic flax oil

3 tablespoons sesame seeds

- Combine all ingredients in a mixing bowl and whisk vigorously, or place ingredients in a blender or food processor and blend thoroughly.

*MAKES ABOUT 1 CUP*

## Rich and Creamy Cheesy Dressing

*A cheesy dressing without the cheese. An excellent choice for those wishing to avoid dairy products but looking for the taste and consistency of cheese.*

| | |
|---|---|
| 3 tablespoons Barlean's organic flax oil | 2 tablespoons eggless mayonnaise |
| 3 tablespoons extra virgin olive oil | 5 tablespoons water |
| 3 tablespoons lemon juice | dash of Worcestershire sauce (optional) |
| 1 large clove garlic, crushed | dash of cayenne |
| 2 teaspoons sesame or poppy seeds | dash of salt (optional) |
| 2 tablespoons tahini | freshly ground black pepper |

- Measure ingredients into a salad bowl. Whisk until thick and creamy.

*SERVES 4 TO 6 (MAKES ABOUT 1 CUP)*

## Creamy Dijon Dressing

4 ounces firm tofu

1/4 cup Barlean's organic flax oil

1 medium clove garlic, crushed

1 small tomato

2 teaspoons soy sauce or tamari

3 tablespoons water

1/2 teaspoon Dijon mustard

2 1/4 tablespoons rice vinegar

3 tablespoons lemon juice

1 tablespoon apple cider vinegar

1 1-inch chunk onion

1 tablespoon minced chives

2 teaspoons dried dill weed

1/4 teaspoon salt or salt substitute

• Combine all ingredients in a blender or food processor and process to a creamy consistency.
*MAKES 1 1/2 CUPS*

## Tahini Dressing

1 tablespoon Barlean's organic flax oil

1 1/2 tablespoons tahini

3 tablespoons water

1 tablespoon lime juice

1 1-inch chunk red onion

1 tablespoon tamari

• Combine all ingredients in a blender or food processor and process to an even consistency.
*MAKES 1/2 CUP*

## Tahini-Mint Dressing

2 tablespoons tahini

2 cloves garlic, pressed

1 tablespoon dried mint or
  2 tablespoons fresh mint

1/2 cup water

1 tablespoon lemon juice

1 teaspoon white miso

2 tablespoons Barlean's organic flax oil

• Combine all ingredients in a blender or food processor and process until smooth.
*MAKES 3/4 CUP*

## Curried Salad Dressing

*Prepared directly in a salad bowl, just add mixed greens and vegetables of your choice.*

2 tablespoons Barlean's organic flax oil

1 tablespoon lemon juice

1 to 2 tablespoons eggless mayonnaise

1 teaspoon raw honey

1/2 teaspoon curry powder

1/2 teaspoon dried basil or 2 teaspoons fresh basil

1 teaspoon minced scallions

1/4 teaspoon salt or 1/2 teaspoon kelp powder

freshly ground black pepper

• Measure ingredients into a salad bowl. Whisk until thick and creamy.
*SERVES 2 (MAKES ABOUT 1/4 CUP)*

# CHAPTER TWENTY-FOUR

# Salads

## Add vim and vigor to your salads
## with fatty acid-rich oil

### SALADS RECIPE INDEX

### FLAX FOR THOUGHT

Salads are generally referred to as healthy, but commercially prepared salads may contain ingredients that include the bad "funny fats" (hydrogenated oils). In addition, commercially available salad dressings almost always use highly refined oils as their primary ingredient. The result is that salads are not nearly as healthful as they could be. By preparing salads at home and using flax oil as an ingredient in place of less healthful oils, you can significantly boost the levels of essential fatty acids in your diet while restricting less healthful fats and oils.

Another benefit of adding flax oil to your favorite salad recipes is that the essential fatty acids cause a feeling of fullness and lasting satisfaction following their ingestion. This phenomenon may limit the calories consumed at a sitting—aiding in diet, weight loss, or maintenance programs. In this way, a salad prepared with flax oil and eaten with one of the soups in Chapter 25 could be experienced as a complete, healthful, and satisfying meal.

---

### Brown Rice and Spinach Salad

*Hearty and healthy.*

2 teaspoons extra virgin olive oil

1 tablespoon minced scallions

4 cups chopped fresh spinach

2 tablespoons Barlean's organic flax oil

2 teaspoons lemon juice

2 teaspoons rice vinegar

2 tablespoons soy sauce or tamari

4 cups cooked brown rice

- Heat the olive oil in a skillet. Add the scallions and sauté until soft, adding a few teaspoons of water to prevent browning. Add the spinach and braise until soft. Set aside.
- In large bowl, combine the flax oil, lemon juice, rice vinegar, and soy sauce. Stir in the rice and the spinach mixture.

*SERVES 4*

---

### Marinated Cauliflower Salad

*A perfect harmony of cruciferous vegetables.*

**Salad**

1 large head cauliflower, cored and sliced

1 cup sliced green olives

1 green bell pepper, cut into thin strips

1 medium onion, chopped

1/4 cup or 2 ounces finely chopped pimentos

**Marinade**

1/4 cup Barlean's organic flax oil

juice of 1/2 lemon

3 tablespoons white wine vinegar

2 teaspoons salt or salt substitute

1/2 teaspoon raw honey

1/4 teaspoon black pepper

- Combine the salad ingredients in a large bowl.
- Mix together the marinade ingredients and pour over the salad. Refrigerate overnight.

*SERVES 4*

## Fruit Salad with Flax-Maple Dressing

1 fresh pineapple, cut into 1-inch pieces

2 golden delicious apples, pared,
cored, and sliced

1 ripe pear, pared, cored, and sliced

1 banana, sliced

1 cup sliced strawberries

2 tablespoons Barlean's organic flax oil

2 tablespoons pure maple syrup

1/4 cup apple juice

1/4 cup chopped pitted dates (optional)

1/4 cup golden raisins (optional)

romaine lettuce leaves

plain nonfat yogurt to top (optional)

- Combine the pineapple, apples, pear, banana, and strawberries in a bowl.
- In another bowl, combine the flax oil, maple syrup, and apple juice and whisk to an even consistency. Add the dates and raisins.
- Combine the two mixtures. Toss lightly to moisten all of the fruit pieces. Cover and refrigerate for 30 minutes.
- When ready to serve, line a salad bowl with the lettuce leaves and arrange the salad on top.
- If desired, top with yogurt.

*SERVES 4*

## Tuna Salad Supreme

*Packed with protein and rich in essential fatty acids.*

1 6 1/4-ounce can water-packed,
no-salt tuna, drained

1 scallion, chopped

2 red radishes, sliced

1 stalk celery, chopped

1 tablespoon no-salt mustard

1 tablespoon Barlean's organic flax oil

1/8 teaspoon cayenne

- Place tuna in a medium bowl and cover with scallion, radishes, celery, mustard, flax oil, and cayenne. Mix together well.
- Serve with a sprig of parsley or use as a sandwich spread.

*SERVES 1 TO 2*

*This recipe comes compliments of* The Fat Burning Diet, *authored by fitness expert Mr. Jay Robb.*

## Mediterranean Salad

1 cucumber, sliced

1 bunch radishes, trimmed

1 red bell pepper, cut into strips

1 green bell pepper, cut into wedges

3 tomatoes, cut into wedges

1/2 bunch chicory or curly endive lettuce, shredded

6 scallions, sliced

3 tablespoons Oregano Dressing (page 144)

2 tablespoons crumbled feta cheese

- In a medium bowl, combine the cucumber, radishes, bell peppers, tomatoes, chicory or lettuce, and scallions. Add the Oregano Dressing and toss to coat well.
- Sprinkle with feta cheese.

*SERVES 4*

## Hearty Vegetable Salad

1 tablespoon Barlean's organic flax oil

1/2 cup red wine vinegar

1/3 cup chopped fresh parsley

2 tablespoons lemon juice

1 clove garlic, minced

2 teaspoons dried basil, crumbled

3/4 teaspoon salt or salt substitute

1/4 teaspoon freshly ground pepper

3 large boiling potatoes, peeled, cooked, and thinly sliced

1 1/2 pounds baby carrots, cooked

1 1/2 pounds green beans, cooked and cut to same length as carrots

3 beets, cooked and thinly sliced

lettuce leaves

- Mix together the flax oil, vinegar, parsley, lemon juice, garlic, basil, salt, and pepper.
- Place the potatoes, carrots, and beans in one bowl and the beets in a smaller bowl. Pour the vinaigrette over the vegetables and stir gently.
- Cover and let marinate for 3 hours at room temperature or refrigerate overnight.
- When ready to serve, line a platter with the lettuce leaves and arrange the vegetables on top.

*SERVES 6*

## Avocado, Jicama, and Grapefruit Salad

*A colorful array of fruit and vegetables that are pleasing to the eye and palate.*

1 large or 2 small avocados

2 medium ruby red grapefruit

1/2 pound jicama

2 tablespoons Barlean's organic flax oil

1 tablespoon minced fresh parsley

- Peel the avocados and cut into wedges. Peel the grapefruit and cut into sections, reserving the juice. Peel the jicama and cut into thin wedges the same length as the avocado slices.
- On 4 individual plates, alternate slices of avocado, grapefruit, and jicama and arrange in a circle or fan.
- Combine the flax oil, reserved grapefruit juice, and parsley in a small bowl. Drizzle over the salads.

*SERVES 4*

## Lentil Salad

1 cup dried lentils

2 quarts water

1 bay leaf

1 clove garlic, minced

1 teaspoon salt or salt substitute

1/4 cup scallions

1/2 cup chopped fresh parsley

1 teaspoon prepared mustard

1/2 teaspoon black pepper

1 tablespoon Barlean's organic flax oil

1 tablespoon lemon juice

1/2 cup grated carrot for garnish

- Clean the lentils and place in a large pot with the water, bay leaf, garlic, and salt. Heat to boiling. Turn the heat off and let sit for 30 minutes. Drain and remove the bay leaf.
- Transfer to a bowl. Add the scallions, parsley, mustard, pepper, flax oil, and lemon juice and mix thoroughly.
- Garnish with grated carrot.

*SERVES 4*

### Rice, Bean, and Corn Salad

*This extremely nutritious and hearty salad can be used as an entrée, especially during the hot summer months.*

2 cups cooked brown rice

1 16-ounce can or 2 cups cooked
red kidney beans, drained and rinsed

1½ cups cooked fresh corn or
thawed frozen corn

4 scallions, chopped

⅛ cup Barlean's organic flax oil

⅛ cup lime juice

⅛ cup cider vinegar

1 tablespoon brown sugar

2 fresh or pickled jalapeño peppers, minced

1 teaspoon chili powder

½ teaspoon ground cumin

½ teaspoon salt or salt substitute

wedges of lime

- Mix together and serve with lime wedges.

*SERVES 4*

### Divine Carrot-Currant Salad

*As a side dish or main meal, this sweet carrot salad is sure to please.*

½ cup currants

½ cup boiling water

2 tablespoons tahini

2 tablespoons Barlean's organic flax oil

1 tablespoon lemon juice

2 teaspoons raw honey

dash of cinnamon

½ cup grated carrot

- Soak the currants in the boiling water for 1 or more hours. Drain and reserve the currant water.
- Combine the currant water, tahini, flax oil, lemon juice, honey, and cinnamon in a food processor or blender and process until creamy.
- Place the carrot and currants in a bowl. Pour the dressing over the salad and mix well.

*SERVES 2*

## Zucchini and Caper Salad

*This is a great summer salad for using the abundance of fresh zucchini produced in a home garden.*

4 large zucchini, quartered lengthwise,
   then cut into 1/2-inch slices

1 small red bell pepper, seeded and
   finely chopped

2 tablespoons capers, rinsed

1 tablespoon chopped fresh parsley

1 tablespoon Barlean's organic flax oil

1 tablespoon lemon juice

1/2 teaspoon dry mustard

1/4 teaspoon black pepper

1 head red leaf lettuce, leaves separated

- In a medium bowl, combine the zucchini, bell pepper, capers, and parsley.
- In a small bowl, combine the flax oil, lemon juice, mustard, and pepper and blend thoroughly.
- Pour the dressing over the zucchini mixture and toss to coat well.
- Line 4 individual serving bowls with the lettuce. Place the zucchini mixture in the centers just before the salads are to be served.

*SERVES 4*

## Caesar Salad

1/2 clove garlic, crushed

3 tablespoons Barlean's organic flax oil

1/2 teaspoon dry mustard

1 tablespoon lemon juice

1 tablespoon white wine vinegar

2 teaspoons soy sauce or tamari

6 Greek olives, pitted and chopped into a paste

2 bunches romaine lettuce, washed, dried,
   and torn into bite-size pieces

1 cup whole-grain croutons

- In a jar with a tight fitting lid, combine the garlic, flax oil, mustard, lemon juice, vinegar, soy sauce, and olive paste. Secure the lid and shake until the dressing is emulsified.
- Place the lettuce in a large salad bowl and toss with the dressing. Sprinkle with croutons and serve immediately.

*SERVES 4*

---

## Vegetable Rice Salad

*This delicious and spicy salad works very well with Indian and East Asian dishes.*

### Salad

2 cups cooked long-grain brown rice

1/4 cup finely sliced radish (about 3 large radishes)

1/2 cup peeled, seeded, and finely diced cucumber

1/2 cup finely diced red bell pepper

1/4 cup finely diced celery

1/4 cup thinly sliced scallions

### Dressing

2 tablespoons extra virgin olive oil

2 tablespoons Barlean's organic flax oil

1/4 cup freshly grated Parmesan cheese

3 tablespoons cider vinegar

2 tablespoons plain nonfat yogurt

1 tablespoon minced fresh basil, or other fresh herb

1/2 teaspoon prepared mustard

### Garnish

lettuce leaves

tomato wedges

2 tablespoons pumpkin seeds (optional)

- Combine all of the salad ingredients in a large bowl.
- Blend all of the dressing ingredients in a small mixing bowl.
- Add the dressing to the salad and mix well. Cover tightly and refrigerate overnight.
- When ready to serve, arrange the lettuce leaves on a large serving platter. Toss the salad lightly and mound it in the center. Garnish with tomato wedges. Sprinkle with pumpkin seeds if desired.

*SERVES 6*

## Taco Salad

*Dressing*

1/4 green bell pepper, very finely chopped

1 scallion, finely chopped

2 tablespoons finely chopped cilantro

3 tablespoons Barlean's organic flax oil

1 tablespoon white vinegar

1 tablespoon lemon juice

1/4 teaspoon salt

1/4 teaspoon chili powder

1/2 clove garlic, crushed

*Salad*

1 head green leaf lettuce, washed and broken into bite-size pieces

1/4 cup sliced black olives

1 tomato, diced

1/2 cup broken tortilla chips or corn chips

*Toppings*

guacamole

6 whole black olives

- Combine the dressing ingredients in a small bowl. Whisk and allow to sit for 30 minutes.
- In a large salad bowl, mix the salad ingredients. Cover with the dressing and toss.
- Serve in large individual salad dishes. Place a generous dab of guacamole on top and garnish with a whole black olive.

*SERVES 6*

## Tabouli

*A zesty and healthful Middle Eastern grain dish.*

1 cup bulgur wheat

2 cups boiling water

2 tomatoes, finely diced

1 bunch scallions with tops, finely chopped

1 cup finely chopped fresh parsley

3 tablespoons chopped fresh mint leaves or 2 teaspoons dried mint

1/4 cup lemon juice

2 tablespoons Barlean's organic flax oil

1/4 teaspoon black pepper

1/4 teaspoon dried oregano

1/4 teaspoon ground cumin

1/4 teaspoon allspice

1/4 teaspoon coriander

- Place the bulgur in a medium bowl and pour the boiling water over the bulgur. Let soak for 1 hour.
- Drain well, pressing out the excess water through a fine strainer or cheesecloth.
- Add the tomatoes, scallions, parsley, and mint to the bulgur and mix thoroughly. Set aside.
- In a small bowl, combine the lemon juice, flax oil, pepper, oregano, cumin, allspice, and coriander.
- Pour the dressing over the bulgur mixture and toss to coat well. Marinate for 1 hour before serving.

*SERVES 6*

---

## Corn Salad

2 24-ounce bags frozen corn

8 ounces Monterey jack or soy cheese, diced

1 large red bell pepper, diced

1 large green bell pepper, diced

1 red onion, diced

3 tablespoons Barlean's organic flax oil

3 tablespoons white wine vinegar

1 tablespoon ground cumin

1 teaspoon salt or salt substitute

1/2 teaspoon black pepper

1/8 teaspoon cayenne

- Cook corn according to package directions. Drain and rinse with cold water.
- Place in a large bowl. Add the cheese, bell peppers, and onion. Toss well.
- Combine the flax oil, vinegar, cumin, salt, pepper, and cayenne in a jar with a tight fitting lid. Shake well.
- Pour the dressing over the corn mixture and mix well. Cover and refrigerate at least 3 hours (or overnight), stirring occasionally.

*SERVES 6*

---

## Waldorf Salad

*This is a fantastic salad, from both taste and nutritional perspectives.*

**Dressing**

10 ounces firm tofu

1/2 cup plain nonfat yogurt

3 tablespoons raw honey

2 tablespoons Barlean's organic flax oil

2 tablespoons lemon juice

juice of 1 orange

1/2 teaspoon ground cloves, cinnamon, nutmeg, or cardamom

1/4 teaspoon vanilla extract (optional)

**Salad**

2 apples, chopped

2 pears, chopped

4 stalks celery, chopped

1/2 cup raisins

- In a blender or food processor, process all of the dressing ingredients until smooth and creamy. The dressing may be refrigerated for up to a week. (Makes about 2 cups of dressing.)
- Mix the salad ingredients together and toss with the dressing. Serve chilled.

*SERVES 4*

CHAPTER TWENTY-FIVE

# Sauces and Soups

## Boosting the nutritional value of sauces and soups the flax way

### SAUCES AND SOUPS RECIPE INDEX

### FLAX FOR THOUGHT

Most of the sauces and soups you find on grocery store shelves contain some form of fat for flavor and texture. Unfortunately, the fats and oils they contain are either highly saturated or health-robbing hydrogenated oils. On the other hand, the no-fat and low-fat brands are completely devoid of the essential good fats and lack the flavor and texture that fats and oils bring to sauces and soups. The solution to obtaining truly healthful sauces and soups is to make them from scratch with flax oil, which will impart greater taste satisfaction and satiety.

Here are some simple improvisations for adding flax oil to sauces and soups.

• Replace less healthful oils in your favorite sauce and soup recipes with an equal amount of flax oil, stirring it in after the sauce or soup has been heated or cooked. If the taste of flax oil is too strong for you, use 1/2 extra virgin olive oil and 1/2 flax oil. (I recommend extra virgin olive oil because it is not subjected to the damaging manufacturing practices common to other grocery store oils.)

- If you are not a cook, you can easily incorporate flax oil into premade sauces and soups by simply stirring some in after the sauce or soup has been heated or cooked. It's a good way to get your flax on the run.

## Sesame Sauce

*An uncooked sauce perfect over pasta or grains.*

1/2 cup sesame seeds

1 teaspoon minced garlic

1/2 teaspoon peeled and crushed fresh ginger (crush through a garlic press)

3 tablespoons Barlean's organic flax oil

3 tablespoons extra virgin olive oil

1 teaspoon sesame oil

1/8 teaspoon red pepper flakes

6 tablespoons soy sauce or tamari

1 tablespoon powdered vegetable broth

1/2 cup water

- Lightly toast the sesame seeds for 1 minute in a frying pan.
- In a blender or food processor, combine the ingredients in descending order, processing after every 3 additions. Process the entire mixture until thick.

*MAKES 1 3/4 CUPS*

## Sweet and Sour Sauce

*Excellent when coupled with brown rice and mixed vegetables.*

2 tablespoons Barlean's organic flax oil

2 tablespoons ketchup or tomato sauce

1/4 cup water

1 tablespoon soy sauce or tamari

1 tablespoon vinegar

2 teaspoons raw honey

2 teaspoons arrowroot

- Combine all ingredients and whisk or blend thoroughly.

*MAKES ABOUT 1/2 CUP*

### Mushroom Stroganoff

*Excellent over pasta. Try over whole grains, too!*

1 tablespoon extra virgin olive oil

1 medium onion, chopped (about 1½ cups)

1 medium clove garlic, crushed

½ pound mushrooms, thinly sliced
(about 4 cups)

3 tablespoons lemon juice

½ teaspoon dried tarragon

½ teaspoon paprika

freshly ground black pepper

¾ cup vegetable broth or water

1 tablespoon tahini

2 tablespoons Barlean's organic flax oil

1 small tomato, peeled, seeded, and diced (optional)

- Heat the olive oil in a skillet. Add the onion and garlic and sauté until soft. Add the mushrooms and sauté until the mushrooms soften. Add the lemon juice, tarragon, paprika, and pepper. Mix well.
- Blend the vegetable broth and tahini. Pour over the mushroom mixture and mix well.
- Remove from heat. Add the flax oil and tomato and stir until an even consistency is achieved.

*SERVES 2*

### Flax Gravy

*Great over mashed potatoes. A creamy gravy with no compromise.*

3 cups potato water or water

2 tablespoons powdered vegetable broth
or 2 vegetable bouillon cubes

3 cups whole wheat flour

3 tablespoons Barlean's organic flax oil

- Heat the water in a pot, whisking in the vegetable broth or bouillon cubes until dissolved.
- Slowly whisk in the flour, over medium-high heat, stirring until gravy thickens to desired consistency.
- Remove from heat and cool to serving temperature.
- Stir in the flax oil and serve.

*MAKES 3 CUPS*

―――⬧―――⬧―――

## Onion Sauce

*A wonderful complement to freshly steamed veggies, a perfect butter-free dip for artichokes, and a winner with broccoli.*

2 tablespoons extra virgin olive oil

1 medium white onion, thinly sliced
  (1 cup packed)

1/4 teaspoon ground thyme

1 cup water

4 teaspoons powdered vegetable broth or miso,
  or 1 vegetable bouillon cube

2 tablespoons Barlean's organic flax oil

- Heat the olive oil in a skillet. Add the onion and thyme. Sauté, stirring for 3 to 4 minutes, until the onion begins to brown. Add the water and powdered vegetable broth, miso, or bouillon cube. Bring to a boil and simmer 3 to 4 minutes over high heat.
- Puree in a blender or food processor. Add the flax oil and blend briefly to combine.

*MAKES 1 1/2 CUPS*

―――⬧―――⬧―――

## Onion Gravy with Tarragon

1 tablespoon extra virgin olive oil

1 large onion, sliced

1 1/2 cups water

2 teaspoons powdered vegetable broth
  or 1 vegetable bouillon cube

1/4 teaspoon dried tarragon

1/4 teaspoon dried sage

1/4 teaspoon dried chervil

dash of nutmeg

2 tablespoons Barlean's organic flax oil

- Heat the olive oil in a medium pan over high heat. Add the onion and sauté, stirring frequently, until the onion is browned. Stir in the water and powdered broth or bouillon cube. Add the tarragon, sage, chervil, and nutmeg. Bring to a boil, lower heat to medium, and simmer gravy until liquid is reduced.
- Remove from heat and cool to serving temperature.
- Stir in the flax oil and serve.

*MAKES ABOUT 2 CUPS*

## Creamy Mushroom-Onion Gravy

*Can't be beat over mashed potatoes or your favorite whole grains.*

| | |
|---|---|
| 1 tablespoon extra virgin olive oil | 3 tablespoons nutritional yeast (optional) |
| 1 white onion, diced | 1¹/₂ cups potato water or water |
| 1 small clove garlic, crushed | 1¹/₂ tablespoons powdered vegetable broth |
| 1 cup sliced mushrooms | or 2 vegetable bouillon cubes |
| 1 tablespoon whole wheat flour | 2¹/₂ tablespoons Barlean's organic flax oil |

- Heat the olive oil in a medium pot. Add the onion and garlic and sauté until soft, about 3 to 4 minutes. Add the mushrooms and sauté 2 to 3 minutes longer, stirring occasionally. Stir in the flour and yeast. Slowly add the water, stirring with a whisk to dissolve lumps until smooth. Add the vegetable broth or crumbled bouillon cubes and continue to stir. Allow gravy to simmer and thicken over medium heat for 5 minutes.
- Remove from heat and cool to serving temperature.
- Stir in the flax oil and serve.

*MAKES 2¹/₂ CUPS*

## Southwestern Sauce

*Inspired by the flavors of New Mexico. Try as a chip dip, taco sauce, or over enchiladas.*

| | |
|---|---|
| 2 tablespoons lemon juice | ¹/₄ teaspoon salt or salt substitute |
| ¹/₂ cup green chilies, braised in oven | ¹/₂ teaspoon ground cumin |
| ¹/₄ cup rice vinegar | 2 tablespoons Barlean's organic flax oil |
| ¹/₂ cup water | 1 teaspoon raw honey |
| 3 tablespoons nutritional yeast | |

- Combine all ingredients in a blender or food processor and process to an even consistency.

*MAKES 1¹/₄ CUPS*

## Spicy Cauliflower Sauce

*A perfect complement to Mexican dishes, especially delicious over enchiladas.*

| | |
|---|---|
| 1 medium cauliflower, chopped | 1 jalapeño pepper |
| ¹/₂ cup (packed) fresh cilantro leaves | 1 teaspoon soy sauce or tamari |
| 2 cloves garlic | 1 cup water |
| 2 tablespoons Barlean's organic flax oil | |

- Steam the cauliflower until tender, about 15 minutes.
- Place the cauliflower in a blender or food processor with the remaining ingredients. Puree until creamy.
- Serve hot.

*MAKES 2 CUPS*

## Szechwan Peanut Sauce

*Delicious over pasta and grains, or use as a dip for vegetables or spring rolls.*

1 medium clove garlic, crushed

1 teaspoon minced fresh ginger
  or 1/2 teaspoon dried ginger

1 tablespoon minced scallions

6 tablespoons peanut butter

2 tablespoons soy sauce or tamari

2 tablespoons raw honey

1 teaspoon dry mustard

1 tablespoon barbecue sauce

2 tablespoons Barlean's organic flax oil

1/3 cup vegetable stock or water

• Combine all ingredients in a food processor or blender and process to desired consistency.
*MAKES ABOUT 1 CUP*

## Pumpkin Seed–Mint Sauce

*Delicious over your favorite grains or vegetables.*

2 tablespoons mayonnaise or eggless mayonnaise

1 cup hot water

1/4 cup pumpkin seeds, toasted lightly

2 large green serrano chilies, seeded and chopped

1/2 teaspoon onion powder

1/2 teaspoon salt or salt substitute

2 tablespoons dried mint
  or 3 tablespoons fresh mint

3 cloves garlic, crushed

3 tablespoons Barlean's organic flax oil

freshly ground black pepper to taste

• Combine all ingredients in a blender or food processor and process until creamy.
*MAKES ABOUT 1 1/2 CUPS*

## No-Cream of Broccoli Soup

1 medium onion, sliced

1 medium carrot, sliced

1 stalk celery, sliced

1 clove garlic

1 cup vegetable broth or water

2 cups chopped broccoli

1/2 cup macaroni

1 cup soy milk, rice milk, or nonfat milk

1/8 teaspoon cayenne

1/8 teaspoon peeled and grated fresh ginger

1/2 teaspoon salt or salt substitute

2 tablespoons Barlean's organic flax oil

• In a covered pot, simmer the onion, carrot, celery, garlic, and vegetable broth for 5 minutes.
• Add the broccoli and macaroni and simmer another 5 to 10 minutes.
• Transfer to a blender. Add the milk, cayenne, ginger, salt, and flax oil and puree.
*SERVES 4*

———◦◦◦———

### Gazpacho

*A chilled soup referred to by many as the "Spanish salad soup."*

| | |
|---|---|
| 1 large onion, chopped | freshly ground black pepper |
| 2 large cloves garlic, crushed | 1 cucumber |
| 1 28-ounce can tomatoes | 1 small green or red bell pepper |
| 3 tablespoons Barlean's organic flax oil | 1 tablespoon chopped fresh chives |
| 2 teaspoons wine vinegar | 1 tablespoon chopped fresh mint |
| 1 1/2 teaspoons salt or substitute | croutons to top |

- Place the onion, garlic, tomatoes, flax oil, vinegar, salt, and a grinding of pepper in a blender or food processor and puree.
- Refrigerate about 2 hours.
- Just before serving the soup, peel the cucumber and remove the seeds from the bell pepper. Chop both into small pieces and stir into the soup, along with the freshly chopped herbs.
- Ladle into individual bowls. Top with croutons.

*SERVES 4*

———◦◦◦———

### Tomato Soup

| | |
|---|---|
| 3 cups finely chopped fresh tomatoes | 3/4 teaspoon dried oregano |
| 1 medium onion, finely chopped | 1 1/2 teaspoons dried basil |
| 2 stalks celery, finely chopped | 2 tablespoons Barlean's organic flax oil |
| 1 large carrot, grated | freshly ground black pepper to taste |
| 1 quart vegetable stock or water | |

- Place the tomatoes, onion, celery, carrot, and vegetable stock in a soup pot. Bring to a boil, then reduce the heat to medium-low. Add the oregano and basil and simmer until the vegetables are tender.
- Remove from heat and stir in the flax oil. Season with pepper.

*SERVES 4*

### Barley Vegetable Soup

*A hearty soup, especially warming after outdoor activity on a brisk fall day.*

| | |
|---|---|
| 1/4 cup washed whole barley | 2 cups skinned and chopped tomatoes |
| 6 cups boiling water | 1 cup peas (fresh or frozen) |
| 1 cup sliced carrots | 3 tablespoons Barlean's organic flax oil |
| 1/2 cup diced celery | 1/2 cup chopped fresh parsley |
| 1/4 cup chopped onion | salt or salt substitute to taste |

- Place the barley and water in a heavy kettle. Cover and simmer until the barley is tender, about 1 hour.
- Add the remaining ingredients, except the flax oil and parsley. Cover and cook until the vegetables are barely tender.
- Remove from heat and stir in the flax oil and parsley. Season to taste.

*SERVES 6*

### Spinach and Parsnip Soup

| | |
|---|---|
| 2 cups water | 1 tablespoon curry powder |
| 3 medium parsnips, chopped | 1 teaspoon dried chervil |
| 1 small onion, chopped | 1/2 teaspoon cinnamon |
| 1 bunch fresh spinach, finely chopped, | 1/4 cup chopped fresh parsley |
| or 10-ounce package frozen chopped spinach | 2 tablespoons Barlean's organic flax oil |
| 1 cup chopped mushrooms | |

- In a soup pot, cook the parsnips and onion in the water until very tender.
- Mash or puree in a blender.
- Return to heat. If the mixture is too thick, add more water.
- In a saucepan, cook the spinach and mushrooms until very tender.
- Mash or puree in a blender, then pour into the parsnip mixture.
- Add the herbs and spices. Stir in the flax oil and serve.

*SERVES 4*

## Carrot and Parsnip Soup with Vegetables

6 medium carrots, chopped

1 large parsnip, chopped

1 small onion, chopped

2 cloves garlic, minced

3 cups water

1 cup chopped broccoli

1 cup chopped asparagus

1 cup chopped zucchini

1 cup peas (fresh or frozen)

1 sprig fresh parsley, finely chopped

1 teaspoon ground cumin

1 teaspoon dried sweet marjoram

1 teaspoon dried basil

1/2 teaspoon white pepper

4 tablespoons Barlean's organic flax oil

- In a soup pot, cook the carrots, parsnip, onion, and garlic in the water until very tender.
- Mash, or transfer to a blender or food processor and puree.
- Return to medium heat, adding water if the mixture is too thick. Add the remaining ingredients, except the flax oil, and cook until tender, but not mushy.
- Remove from heat and stir in the flax oil.

*SERVES 6*

## Sweet Potato–Pumpkin Soup

1/2 quart peeled sweet potatoes, cut into chunks

1/2 quart peeled pumpkin, cut into chunks

3 cups thickly sliced leeks or onions

3 carrots, cut into chunks

3 stalks celery, cut into large chunks

2 quarts water

1 teaspoon salt or salt substitute

1/2 teaspoon freshly ground pepper

2 tablespoons toasted sesame seeds

1 tablespoon caraway seeds

2 tablespoons chopped fresh tarragon
  or 1/2 teaspoon dried tarragon

4 tablespoons Barlean's organic flax oil

- Place the sweet potatoes, pumpkin, leeks or onions, carrots, celery, water, salt, and pepper in a large kettle. Bring to a boil, then cover and simmer for 40 minutes. The soup will be lumpy.
- With a slotted spoon, remove and reserve half of the carrots and celery and some firmer potato chunks.
- Puree the remainder of the soup in a food mill or blender until smooth.
- Return to the kettle and add the sesame seeds, caraway seeds, tarragon, and the reserved vegetables. Stir in the flax oil and serve.

*SERVES 8*

## Lentil Soup

1 tablespoon extra virgin olive oil

2 large onions, finely diced

4 cloves garlic, crushed or minced

2 green bell peppers, finely diced

10 cups vegetable stock

2 carrots, thinly sliced

1 1/2 cups lentils

1/3 teaspoon dried thyme

liberal seasoning with freshly ground black pepper

1/2 teaspoon salt or salt substitute

1 28-ounce can plum tomatoes in their juice, finely chopped

1 pound fresh spinach, stems removed and finely chopped, or 10-ounce package frozen chopped spinach, thawed

4 tablespoons Barlean's organic flax oil

- Heat the olive oil in a large stock pot over medium heat. Add the onions, garlic, and bell peppers and sauté for 10 minutes.
- Add the remaining ingredients, except the spinach and flax oil, and bring to a boil. Reduce the heat and simmer, stirring occasionally, for 45 minutes or until the lentils are tender.
- Add the spinach and cook for 5 minutes, or until the spinach has wilted and become tender.
- Remove from heat and stir in the flax oil.

*SERVES 6*

## Curried Red Lentil Soup

1 1/2 cups red lentils

4 cups water

1/2 teaspoon salt or salt substitute

2 medium potatoes, diced

1 tablespoon extra virgin olive oil

1 medium onion, chopped

2 cloves garlic, minced

1 teaspoon turmeric

1 teaspoon ground cumin

1 teaspoon ground coriander

1/2 teaspoon cayenne

2 to 3 tablespoons Barlean's organic flax oil

- Place the lentils in a strainer and rinse with cold, running water.
- Combine the lentils, water, and salt in a large pot. Bring to a boil and cook, uncovered, for 20 minutes over medium heat, stirring occasionally.
- Add the potatoes and stir.
- In a small skillet, heat the olive oil. Add the onion, garlic, and spices. Sauté until the onion begins to get tender.
- Add the onion mixture to the soup and cook until the potatoes are tender, about 20 minutes.
- Remove from heat and stir in the flax oil.

*SERVES 4*

## Black Bean Soup

*This soup can be made up to 4 days ahead: simply pour it into an airtight container, refrigerate, and reheat to serving temperature.*

2 teaspoons extra virgin olive oil

2 medium red onions, chopped

1 jalapeño pepper, minced

2 large cloves garlic, minced

1 teaspoon ground cumin

1/2 teaspoon chili powder

4 cups cooked black beans

2 cups water

2 tablespoons Barlean's organic flax oil

2 tablespoons sour cream
    or plain nonfat yogurt to top

- Heat the olive oil in a medium saucepan. Add the onions and jalapeño pepper. Sauté over moderate heat, stirring frequently, until the onions begin to brown, about 4 minutes.
- Stir in the garlic and reduce the heat to low. Cook, stirring constantly, for 1 minute. Stir in the cumin and chili powder.
- Combine the onion mixture, beans, and water in a heavy pot. Cook over low heat, stirring occasionally, until the beans are hot, about 5 minutes.
- If a smooth texture is preferred, transfer the soup to a food processor or blender and puree until smooth.
- Once the soup is removed from heat, stir in the flax oil.
- Top with a dollop of sour cream or yogurt.

*SERVES 4*

## Ratatouille Soup

1 pound tomatoes, chopped

1 onion, chopped

1 green bell pepper, chopped

2 cloves garlic, minced

2 bay leaves

tomato juice or water if necessary

1 eggplant, unpeeled and chopped

1 teaspoon dried basil

1 teaspoon dried marjoram

1/2 teaspoon dried oregano

1/2 teaspoon dried rosemary

1/4 cup chopped fresh parsley

3 tablespoons Barlean's organic flax oil

- In a soup pot, cook the tomatoes, onion, bell pepper, garlic, and bay leaves until almost tender. If the mixture is too thick, add tomato juice or water.
- Add the eggplant, basil, marjoram, oregano, and rosemary. Cook until the eggplant and other ingredients are tender.
- Add the parsley and heat through.
- Remove from heat and stir in the flax oil.
- Remove the bay leaves before serving. Serve hot or cold.

*SERVES 4*

---

## Split Green Pea Soup

10 cups vegetable stock or water

2 cups split green peas, rinsed and drained

1 tablespoon extra virgin olive oil

1 large onion, finely chopped

1 stalk celery, finely chopped

1 large carrot, finely chopped

salt or salt substitute to taste

freshly ground black pepper to taste

3 tablespoons Barlean's organic flax oil

- In a large stock pot, bring the stock or water to a boil. Add the split peas. Cover and simmer over low heat for about 30 minutes.
- In a pan, heat the olive oil and add the onion, celery, and carrot. Cover and cook until the vegetables have softened, about 15 minutes.
- Add the softened vegetables to the split peas. Season with salt and pepper. Cover and simmer gently for 45 to 60 minutes, stirring occasionally to prevent the soup from sticking to the pot.
- Transfer to a blender. Add the flax oil and puree. If the soup seems too thick, add more water.

*SERVES 6*

---

## Split Pea Soup

*A warming and nourishing soup.*

5 1/2 cups water

1 1/2 cups split peas, rinsed and drained

1 tablespoon concentrated vegetable stock
    or 1 vegetable bouillon cube

1/2 tablespoon onion powder

1/2 teaspoon dried dill weed
    or 1 tablespoon minced fresh dill

dash of cayenne

1/2 cup chopped green bell pepper

1/2 cup minced carrot

1/2 cup quartered and thinly sliced carrot

3 tablespoons Barlean's organic flax oil

- Bring the water to a boil in a large pot. Stir in the peas with the vegetable stock or bouillon cube. Cover and cook over low heat for 1 hour.
- Add the remaining spices and vegetables. Cover and simmer for 20 to 25 minutes.
- Remove from heat and cool to serving temperature.
- Stir in the flax oil and serve.

*SERVES 6*

# CHAPTER TWENTY-SIX

# Entrées and Vegetable Dishes

*The no, no-fat "weigh" to weight loss*
*and maintenance*

## ENTRÉES AND VEGETABLE DISHES RECIPE INDEX

## FLAX FOR THOUGHT

Entrées are the focal point of our dining experience. We have grown to expect hearty, filling, and satisfying entrées, and so they should be. However, we have also been taught that fat is bad and that fat should be low or nonexistent in our main meals. We know from the introductory chapter to this book that this is really only half the story. Fat in meals causes a sensation of fullness and satisfaction. This feeling of satisfaction and fullness effectively curtails our appetite and stabilizes our blood sugar and energy levels for longer periods compared with meals free of fat.

With the recipes presented in *The Healing Power of Flax* you can experience the best of both worlds by limiting your intake of saturated fats and hydrogenated oils and by including the healing and protective essential fats found in flax oil. Flax oil added to your main meals will bring you the satisfaction you expect without the guilt associated with meals high in fat. The essential fatty acids in flax oil help to activate special fat-burning cells in your body that will, in turn, mobilize and burn the bad fats in your body tissues. Can we eat filling, satisfying meals and still maintain or even reduce our waistline? You bet we can, and the answer is the addition of the essential fatty acids found in flax oil.

Here are a few tips regarding entrées and vegetable dishes.

- Create ways to include flax oil in your entrées. Think of flax oil as a tasty carrier for other herbs and as a natural pick-me-up.
- Flax oil can be used as a delicious sauce over brown rice or freshly steamed vegetables.
- Remember, it is important to add flax oil after the cooking process in order to limit the oil's exposure to heat.

### Angel Hair Pasta with Fresh Tomato Sauce

8 ounces angel hair pasta

3 large beefsteak tomatoes,
   cut into 1/2 -inch cubes

1 large clove garlic, crushed

1/4 cup chopped fresh basil
   or 2 teaspoons dried basil

1/4 teaspoon salt or salt substitute

freshly ground black pepper to taste

2 tablespoons Barlean's organic flax oil

- Prepare the pasta according to directions on package.
- Combine the tomatoes, garlic, basil, salt, and pepper. Add the flax oil and whisk well.
- Add half of the sauce to the hot pasta and mix.
- Top with the remaining sauce.

*SERVES 4*

### Winter Pesto

*The perfect complement to pasta dishes.*

3 cups (tightly packed) fresh spinach leaves,
   rinsed and dried

1 tablespoon dried basil

4 cloves garlic

3 tablespoons extra virgin olive oil

2 tablespoons Barlean's organic flax oil

1/3 cup pine nuts

dash of salt or salt substitute

- Combine all ingredients in a blender or food processor and process until smooth.
- Refrigerate in a tightly sealed container until ready to use.
- Bring the pesto to room temperature before serving.

*SERVES 6*

## Spaghetti with Marinara Sauce

3/4 pound spaghetti

1 tablespoon extra virgin olive oil

3/4 cup chopped onion

1/3 cup chopped celery

1/3 cup chopped carrot

1 medium clove garlic, crushed

1 tablespoon nutritional yeast (optional)

6 large tomatoes, peeled and chopped,
   or 28-ounce can peeled Italian tomatoes,
   drained and chopped

1/4 teaspoon dried oregano

1/4 teaspoon dried basil

pinch of salt or salt substitute to taste

freshly ground black pepper to taste

1 tablespoon tomato paste (optional)

1 tablespoon Barlean's organic flax oil

- Prepare the spaghetti according to directions on package.
- While the spaghetti cooks, prepare the sauce.
- Heat the olive oil in a medium pan. Add the onion, celery, carrot, and garlic. Sauté over medium heat for 3 minutes, stirring frequently. Add the yeast and stir well.
- Add the tomatoes, oregano, basil, salt, and pepper. Stir in the tomato paste. Cover and simmer over low heat, stirring occasionally, until the sauce becomes fairly uniform in consistency, about 20 minutes.
- Remove from heat and stir in the flax oil.
- Pour the sauce over the hot spaghetti.

*SERVES 3*

## Vermicelli Pesto and Green Peas

*A simple and delicious meal complemented with fresh basil.*

1/2 pound vermicelli

2 cloves garlic, crushed

4 cups fresh basil leaves

4 tablespoons pine nuts

pinch of salt

1/4 cup Barlean's organic flax oil

1/4 cup extra virgin olive oil

2 cups green peas

- Prepare the pasta according to directions on package.
- While the pasta cooks, prepare the pesto. In a food processor or blender, combine the garlic, basil leaves, pine nuts, salt, flax and olive oils and process to a thick paste.
- Place the peas in a steamer and steam for 4 to 5 minutes or until tender.
- Remove 1/2 cup of the pasta water from pot before draining the pasta. Combine the pasta water with 1/4 cup of the pesto and stir well. (Store the remaining pesto.*)
- Place the pasta in a large bowl. Add the peas and pour the pesto over the top. Toss well.

* *Note: Cover the remaining pesto with a thin layer of olive oil to prevent the basil leaves from turning brown. Refrigerate. Will keep for several weeks.*

*SERVES 2*

~~~~~~

### Peanut Butter, Flax, and Carrot Sandwich

*Packed with punch for a high-energy lunch.*

1 tablespoon Barlean's organic flax oil

2 tablespoons natural peanut butter

2 slices whole-grain bread

1/4 cup shredded baby carrots

lettuce or alfalfa sprouts

- Combine the flax oil and peanut butter. Stir to an even consistency.
- Spread both pieces of bread with the flax–peanut butter mixture. Add the carrots and lettuce or sprouts.
- Eat!

*SERVES 1*

~~~~~~

### Whipped Acorn Squash and Yams

*A twist on tradition by adding flax oil.*

2 large acorn squash, halved

2 large or 4 medium yams

1/2 cup fresh orange juice

1 tablespoon pure maple syrup

cinnamon

grated nutmeg

3 tablespoons Barlean's organic flax oil

- Bake the squash and yams for 45 minutes to 1 hour or until tender.
- Scoop out the squash from the skins and place in a large mixing bowl or food processor. Remove the yam flesh from the skins and add to the squash.
- Add the orange juice, maple syrup, spices, and flax oil. Whip or mash together.

*SERVES 6*

~~~~~~

### Corn on the Cob with Spicy Flax Sauce

*A tastier and healthier alternative to butter for delicious corn on the cob.*

1/2 teaspoon pressed garlic
  or 1/2 teaspoon garlic powder

1/4 teaspoon ground cumin

1/4 teaspoon paprika

dash of cayenne

2 tablespoons Barlean's organic flax oil

6 ears corn (fresh or frozen)

- Combine the garlic and spices with the flax oil.
- Bring a large pot of water to a boil. Add the corn and return to a boil, then boil for 3 minutes.
- Remove the corn from the water and brush generously with the spicy flax sauce.

*SERVES 6*

## Marinated Artichokes

*This is a great dish to serve while entertaining.*

2 artichokes, cooked

$1^1/2$ teaspoons grated orange peel

$1/2$ cup orange juice

$1/2$ teaspoon salt or salt substitute

$1/8$ cup Barlean's organic flax oil

pinch of each: tarragon, basil, and chervil

2 tablespoons tarragon vinegar

$1/4$ teaspoon dry mustard

2 tablespoons chopped shallot or scallions

$1/4$ teaspoon Worcestershire sauce

1 tablespoon minced fresh parsley

- Cut the artichokes in half from tip to stem. Remove and discard the choke and the small inner leaves.
- Combine the remaining ingredients in a food processor or blender and process to an even consistency.
- Place the artichokes in a shallow dish and spoon the marinade over them. Cover and refrigerate overnight, turning occasionally.
- Serve the artichokes with some of the marinade spooned over the top.

*SERVES 2*

## Marinated Roasted Red Peppers

4 large red bell peppers

2 cloves garlic, crushed or sliced into thin slivers

4 tablespoons Barlean's organic flax oil

$1/2$ teaspoon kelp powder or vegetable seasoning

- Place the peppers on a baking sheet in a preheated 400°F oven. Turn frequently until skin blisters on all sides.
- Remove the peppers from the oven and place in a paper bag. Close tightly. Allow to sit for 20 minutes while the skins sweat off.
- Peel the loose skins from the peppers, remove the seeds and ribs, and discard. Cut the peppers in strips of desired thickness.
- Combine the flax oil, garlic, and kelp powder in a medium bowl.
- Add the pepper strips and marinate at least 1 hour before using, or store in the refrigerator in a tightly sealed container until ready to use.

*SERVES 4*

---

### Barlean's Marinated Red Pepper Sandwich

*Nutritious and delicious.*

2 slices whole-grain bread, lightly toasted
mayonnaise or Flax-Almond
   Mayonnaise (page 137)
Dijon mustard

Marinated Roasted Red Peppers (page 175)
grated carrot
thinly sliced cucumber

- Spread the bread generously with mayonnaise and mustard.
- Add the remaining ingredients.

*SERVES 1*

---

### Sauerkraut Hawaiian Style

*Combines sulfur-rich cruciferous vegetables with fatty acid-rich flax oil.*

8 ounces sauerkraut with liquid
8 ounces red cabbage
1/2 cup diced pineapple

1 cup diced tomatoes
1 teaspoon soy sauce or tamari
2 tablespoons Barlean's organic flax oil

- Combine the sauerkraut with liquid, cabbage, pineapple, and tomatoes in a saucepan. Simmer for 30 minutes.
- Remove from heat and stir in the soy sauce and flax oil.
- Serve hot or cold.

*SERVES 2 TO 3*

# CHAPTER TWENTY-SEVEN

# Desserts and Treats

## *Fun and frolic with flax*

## DESSERTS AND TREATS RECIPE INDEX

### FLAX FOR THOUGHT

Desserts and treats are often considered the downfall of our dining experience. This belief is well founded because the majority of desserts and treats available to us are highly processed and full of refined sugar as well as unnatural saturated fats. How often have we heard "no dessert for me, I'm trying to drop a couple of pounds." An hour later, the well-intentioned diner is downing a half gallon of ice cream from the carton. Is it possible to provide sensible, satisfying, and healthful desserts and treats for your friends, family, and self? Absolutely. And the result will be far healthier than a late-night binge.

As is common with other foods, much of the satisfaction that is found with desserts is because they bring satiety, the sense of fulfillment following a meal. The primary reason for satiety in foods is because of the fat found in them. If you've ever eaten a low-fat or no-fat dessert, you know what I mean. The sweetness might be there, but somehow you are left craving more, so you have another and another and another—you get the idea. Not a bad way to sell more no-fat and low-fat desserts. Unfortunately, as we have learned, you end up eating more calories than if you had just eaten a sensible portion of a dessert or treat that contained some fat—hopefully good fat.

The best news is that we can enjoy delicious, healthful, and satisfying desserts and treats without the guilt associated with highly refined or unhealthfully saturated and funny fat-laden desserts. You will find that by adding flax oil to desserts and treats, you can experience a sense of enjoyment and satisfaction with a single serving and avoid eating seconds and thirds. You will also appreciate the sustained energy and blood sugar levels that flax oil brings, satisfying your hunger for hours on end.

Here are a few suggestions for terrific flax desserts.

- With a little creativity, flax oil can be incorporated into many desserts. Try mixing flax oil half and half with pure maple syrup as a topping. Another option is to mix flax oil half and half with raw honey for a delicious, sweet spread or topping. Try pureeing the oil with your favorite berries in a blender or food processor.
- Spice up your flax oil with a dash of cinnamon, allspice, nutmeg, or other pleasant spice to make flax oil more applicable for use in desserts.
- In recipes that don't require excessive heating or baking, simply replace or reduce the less healthful oils in the recipe with flax oil. Because unrefined flax oil exerts a stronger flavor than refined oils, make sure the nutty flavor of quality flax oil will enhance the recipe.

### Coconut-Mocha Cream Frosting

| | |
|---|---|
| 5 tablespoons whole wheat pastry flour | 3 tablespoons pure maple syrup |
| 1 cup rice milk or soy milk | 1/2 cup shredded coconut |
| 2 tablespoons Barlean's organic flax oil | 1 teaspoon carob powder |
| 1/4 teaspoon salt | 1 teaspoon Pero, Roma, |
| 2 teaspoons vanilla extract | or other powdered coffee substitute |

- In a small saucepan, combine the flour and milk. Bring to a boil, whisking constantly. If lumps appear, beat with an eggbeater until smooth. Stirring constantly, cook until the flour is thickened, about 2 minutes. Cool for 15 minutes.
- Place the flour mixture and the remaining ingredients in a blender and blend at medium speed until very smooth. Cool for 30 minutes. Whisk well before using.

*FROSTS ONE SINGLE-LAYER CAKE*

### Carob-Peanut Butter Bars

| | |
|---|---|
| 1/2 cup carob powder | 2 tablespoons brewers yeast, optional |
| 2/3 cup soy powder | 2 tablespoons wheat germ |
| 2 tablespoons Barlean's organic flax oil | raw honey |
| 1/4 cup peanut butter | chopped walnuts and almonds to top |
| 1/4 cup rice polishings | |

- Place all ingredients in a bowl, adding enough honey to make a kneadable consistency.
- Spread in a square pan. Press the chopped nuts over the top. Chill.
- Cut into bars and serve.

*MAKES 6 BARS*

## Flax, Bran, and Fruit Bars

*A healthy snack alternative.*

1/4 pound pitted dried prunes

1/4 pound dates

1/4 pound figs

1/4 pound raisins

1/4 cup raw honey

3 tablespoons lemon juice

3 tablespoons Barlean's organic flax oil

1 cup bran

1/2 cup wheat germ

1 tablespoon grated orange rind

- Process the fruit in a food processor.
- Combine the honey, lemon juice, flax oil, bran, wheat germ, and orange rind. Mix well.
- Combine the processed fruit with the other ingredients and mix well.
- Mold the mixture in a pan and refrigerate 1 hour.
- Cut into bars and serve.

*MAKES 12 BARS*

## Tofu Yogurt

*If you are allergic to milk or simply desire the nutritional benefits of soy, this is a great alternative to standard yogurt.*

1/2 block silken tofu

1 to 1 1/2 cups frozen and chopped
   strawberries, blueberries, or raspberries

1 tablespoon Barlean's organic flax oil

1 teaspoon vanilla extract

1 teaspoon raw honey

- Combine ingredients in order listed in a food processor or blender and process to an even consistency.

*SERVES 1*

———————

### Peach Pie

1 standard whole wheat piecrust,
  baked to a light brown
5 to 6 large peaches, peeled
3 tablespoons fresh orange juice
1/2 cup raw cashew pieces
3 tablespoons pure maple syrup

1/2 cup water
1 teaspoon vanilla extract
1/2 cup Barlean's organic flax oil
fresh mint leaves for garnish
plain yogurt to top

- Slice the peaches into thin half moons.
- In a mixing bowl, combine the peaches with the orange juice and set aside.
- Place the cashews in a blender or food processor with the maple syrup, water, and vanilla. Process until creamy and smooth. While the blender is running on low speed, add the flax oil in a thin stream until the mixture thickens but is still slightly runny.
- Coat the bottom of the piecrust with a thin layer of the cashew mixture. Add a layer of peach slices in flower petal fashion, then spread with cashew mixture and continue layering, ending with a top layer of peaches. Garnish with mint leaves.
- Refrigerate for at least 2 hours before serving.
- Top with yogurt.

*MAKES 1 PIE*

———————

### Peach Melba

3 peaches, peeled and halved,
  or 6 canned peach halves (juice packed)
6 tablespoons vanilla or plain nonfat yogurt

1 1/2 tablespoons Barlean's organic flax oil
6 tablespoons pureed raspberries

- Place the peach halves in individual sherbet glasses.
- Combine the yogurt and flax oil in a small bowl and stir thoroughly to homogenize.
- Top each peach with 1 tablespoon of the yogurt mixture and then with 1 tablespoon of the pureed raspberries.

*SERVES 6*

## Sautéed Apples with Maple Syrup-Yogurt Topping

*A taste treat. This recipe is also good with pears used in place of apples.*

6 medium apples, peeled and quartered

1 tablespoon butter

5 tablespoons pure maple syrup

1/4 teaspoon ground cloves

1 1/2 teaspoons cinnamon

1 cup plain nonfat yogurt

4 tablespoons Barlean's organic flax oil

2 tablespoons chopped walnuts to top

- Cut each apple quarter into 4 slices.
- Sauté the apples in the butter for 5 minutes. Add 4 tablespoons of the maple syrup, the cloves, and one half of the cinnamon. Stir to coat the apples. Cook about 7 minutes more, until the apples are tender and the syrup thickens.
- Transfer to a medium bowl and chill for 1 hour.
- In another medium bowl, combine the yogurt, the remaining maple syrup and cinnamon, and the flax oil. Stir to an even consistency. Chill for at least 1 hour.
- When ready to serve, place the apple mixture in individual bowls. Spoon the yogurt mixture on top and sprinkle with the walnuts.

*SERVES 6*

## Strawberry-Banana Pie

1 homemade or prepared whole wheat piecrust lightly browned in the oven

### Strawberry Glaze

2 cups strawberries

2 tablespoons psyllium husks
(available in health food stores)

2 tablespoons pure maple syrup

2 tablespoons Barlean's organic flax oil

### Filling

3 medium bananas

3 cups strawberries

shredded coconut to top

- Blend the strawberries, psyllium, maple syrup, and flax oil. Pour two-thirds of the glaze into the crust, reserving one-third for the top.
- Thinly slice the bananas and strawberries. Cover the bottom of the pie first with a layer of half the strawberries, then with the banana slices. Top with a final layer of strawberries and the remainder of the glaze. Sprinkle with coconut.
- Refrigerate at least 3 hours before serving.

*SERVES 6*

---

## Coconut, Carob, and Peanut Butter Balls

*A taste treat better than See's candies. A favorite with kids!*

| | |
|---|---|
| 1/2 cup natural peanut butter | 1/2 cup shredded coconut (more if necessary) |
| 1/2 cup Barlean's organic flax oil | 1/4 cup carob powder |

- In a bowl, combine the peanut butter and flax oil and mix thoroughly.
- Stir in the coconut and carob powder. If necessary, use additional coconut to thicken mixture.
- Form the dough into balls.
- Serve immediately, or cover and chill for future use.

### Variations:

- add 1/4 cup raisins
- add 1/4 cup walnuts

SERVES 6

---

## Spanish Baklava

*By using tortillas instead of filo dough we have come up with a quick and easy south-of-the-border revision of the tasty traditional Middle Eastern treat.*

| | |
|---|---|
| 1/2 cup water | 1 tablespoon raw honey |
| 1/4 cup raisins | 1/4 teaspoon cinnamon |
| 2 flour or whole wheat tortillas | 1/2 cup plain yogurt |
| 2 tablespoons Barlean's organic flax oil | 2 tablespoons crushed walnuts |
| 1 tablespoon pure maple syrup | |

- Heat the water to boiling. Add the raisins. Remove from heat and set aside.
- Heat the tortillas in a frying pan over low heat, maintaining softness and pliability (don't overcook).
- While heating the tortillas, combine the flax oil, maple syrup, honey, and cinnamon in a small bowl and whisk well.
- Pour the raisins into a strainer, discarding the water.
- Remove the tortillas from heat.
- Spread an even layer of the flax oil mixture over the entire face of both tortillas.
- Form a line with the yogurt across the center of the tortillas extending from edge to edge.
- Place the raisins and walnuts over the yogurt.
- Fold the tortillas on both ends and roll tightly (burrito style).
- With a sharp knife make several diagonal cuts in the rolled tortillas.
- Serve immediately, or chill for dessert.

SERVES 6

## Flax Snacks

*An excellent snack between meals. High in dietary fiber.*

3/4 cup flax flour*

3 tablespoons oat flour

1 1/2 teaspoons cinnamon

1 1/2 teaspoons ground cloves

2 tablespoons peanut butter

1/2 cup rice syrup

coconut flakes (optional)

6 tablespoons ground almonds (optional)

* *Grind whole flaxseed to the consistency of flour in a coffee grinder.*

- Combine the flax flour, oat flour, cinnamon, and cloves in a mixing bowl. Add the peanut butter and rice syrup to the mixture. Knead thoroughly by hand.

- Tear pieces off and roll them between your hands into balls. You could also roll the mixture into a log, then cut the log into individual pieces.

- Place the coconut flakes and ground almonds on waxed paper. Press the rolled balls or pieces onto the coconut-almond mixture. (Optional)

- Serve immediately, or chill for future use.

*MAKES ABOUT 2 DOZEN 1-INCH BALLS*

*Recipe submitted by Jo Ann Barlean*

CHAPTER TWENTY-EIGHT

# Flaxy Smoothies

*Flax your muscles with super smoothies*

## FLAXY SMOOTHIES RECIPE INDEX

## FLAX FOR THOUGHT

Of all of the ways presented in *The Healing Power of Flax* to incorporate essential fatty acids into a daily diet, I believe the addition of flax oil to smoothies (blender drinks) is one of the easiest and tastiest ways to get a daily dose of these vital nutrients. In addition, this method lends itself perfectly to the inclusion of a protein source as popularized by Dr. Johanna Budwig, a Nobel Prize nominee, German biochemist, and the world's leading authority on fats and oils nutrition. Dr. Budwig contends that the combination of flax oil with a sulfur-rich protein, such as yogurt or cottage cheese, potentiates the power of the essential fatty acids in the flax oil. Since 1950, Dr. Budwig has treated cancer and other debilitating illnesses with this approach.

You will find these flaxy smoothies to be the perfect midday pick-me-up and, of course, an unbeatable drink after a workout.

Smoothie flax facts:

• Try a smoothie coupled with yogurt, fresh seasonal fruit, and flax oil for a breakfast on the run. You will be amazed at how long this formula will maintain your energy and blood sugar levels.

• Consider adding a scoop of your favorite protein powder or a dollop of yogurt to your smoothies in order to obtain the valuable oil/protein combination endorsed by Dr. Johanna Budwig. This is especially an effective method following a grueling workout. Bodybuilders and fitness buffs have popularized the use of flax oil in smoothies to help reduce the soreness and muscle fatigue associated with training. Jay Robb, a well-known author for bodybuilding magazines and a fat-burning expert, has coined the phrase "flax your muscles" as a testament to these truths.

- For those rare individuals who do not care for the rich taste of unrefined flax oil, the addition of the oil to smoothies goes virtually undetected.
- For those finicky kids, I do not know of a better way to sneak in the benefits of flax oil than through a delicious smoothie.
- Flax oil can be included in any existing smoothie recipe or in any recipe you could dream up.
- Smoothies—a terrific and delicious way to flax your way to good health!

### Banana-Carob Chip Frosty

*A chocolate-like treat.*

2 medium frozen bananas

1 cup frozen rice milk or soy milk (use ice tray)

1 tablespoon peanut butter

¹/₄ cup carob chips

³/₄ cup water

2 tablespoons Barlean's organic flax oil

- In a blender, combine ingredients in order listed and puree to a frosty consistency.

*SERVES 2 TO 3*

### Strawberry and Cashew Nut Milk Smoothie

*Rich, creamy, and nutritious too!*

1³/₄ cups water

¹/₃ cup cashews

7 frozen strawberries

¹/₄ cup frozen blueberries

2 tablespoons Barlean's organic flax oil

2 tablespoons raw honey

- In a blender, combine ingredients in order listed and blend until rich and creamy.

*SERVES 2*

### Pineapple and Cranberry Smoothie

1 cup chunk pineapple

1 medium banana

1 cup cranberry juice

¹/₂ cup plain nonfat yogurt

3 tablespoons raw honey

3 tablespoons Barlean's organic flax oil

2 cups ice (1 tray)

- In a blender, combine ingredients in order listed and puree to a smooth, frosty consistency.

*SERVES 4*

~~~

## Pineapple and Date Smoothie

3/4 cup unsweetened pineapple juice

5 honey dates, pitted

1 frozen banana, sliced

2 tablespoons Barlean's organic flax oil

4 tablespoons plain nonfat yogurt (optional)

3 ice cubes

- In a blender, combine ingredients in order listed and blend until smooth.

SERVES 2

~~~

## Very Cherry Smoothie

*Folkloric belief has established cherries as being beneficial to people suffering from arthritis. The anti-inflammatory action of essential fatty acid-rich flax oil serves to synergise their effect.*

2 cups pitted fresh cherries

1 cup plain nonfat yogurt

2 tablespoons Barlean's organic flax oil

1 tablespoon raw honey

1/4 teaspoon vanilla

1 cup ice (7 ice cubes)

- In a blender, combine ingredients in order listed and puree to a frosty consistency.

*SERVES 2 TO 3*

~~~

## Pineapple-Strawberry Smoothie

1 1/2 cups chilled pineapple juice

2 tablespoons Barlean's organic flax oil

4 tablespoons nonfat yogurt (optional)

10 frozen strawberries

ice cubes

- In a blender, combine ingredients in order listed and puree to a smooth consistency, adding ice cubes as needed.

*SERVES 2*

~~~

## Blueberry-Almond Smoothie

*Refreshing, nourishing, and satisfying.*

1 cup frozen blueberries

1 frozen banana

1/4 cup soft tofu (optional)

1/4 cup raw almonds

2 tablespoons Barlean's organic flax oil

2 tablespoons pure maple syrup

1 cup water or rice milk

- In a blender, combine ingredients in order listed and puree to a smooth consistency.

*SERVES 2*

## Spicy Apple Smoothie

*Rich in fiber and essential fatty acids.*

2 apples, peeled

1 frozen banana

1/4 cup raisins, soaked

1/4 teaspoon peanut butter

2 tablespoons Barlean's organic flax oil

1 tablespoon raw honey

pinch of cinnamon

1 cup water

4 ice cubes

- In a blender, combine all ingredients and puree to a smooth consistency.

*SERVES 2 TO 3*

## Carob Date Shake

*A delectable, chocolatey-tasting, and protein-packed treat!*

2/3 cup water

1 cup soft tofu

2/3 cup honey dates, pitted

1 frozen banana

1 cup crushed ice

2 tablespoons Barlean's organic flax oil

1 tablespoon roasted carob powder
   or cocoa powder

2 teaspoons Pero, Roma,
or other powdered coffee substitute

- In a blender, combine ingredients in order listed. Blend on high speed to desired consistency.

*SERVES 2*

## Nutty Buddy Peanut Butter Smoothie

*A must for the peanut butter lover! A favorite with kids.*

1 cup rice milk, soy milk, or nonfat milk

1 banana

2 tablespoons peanut butter

2 tablespoons raw honey

2 tablespoons plain nonfat yogurt (optional)

2 tablespoons Barlean's organic flax oil

2 tablespoons wheat germ

1/2 teaspoon vanilla

2 cups ice (1 tray)

- In a blender, combine ingredients in order listed and blend until smooth or to desired consistency.

*SERVES 2*

# Resources

The following are the companies I want to tell you about because these are probably the very finest sources of flaxseed oil, milled flaxseed, flax lignans and omega-3 fatty acids today.

**Barlean's Organic Oils**
4936 Lake Terrell Rd.
Ferndale, Washington 98248
(360) 384-0485
www.barleans.com

*Barlean's Organic Oils is producing the finest organic, lignan-rich, unfiltered flax oil today. Besides producing wonderful tasting, unfiltered flax oils, they also produce organic evening primrose, borage and other oil products. Look for their* Essential Woman *and* Omega Man *oil products and flax products for pets. Barlean's has consistently been the recipient of the coveted Vity Award year after year for the quality of its organic oils. (The Vity Awards are the nutrition industry's equivalent to the Emmys or Oscars and voted on by retailers themselves.) I especially recommend their Forti-Flax milled flaxseed and, of course, their Highest Lignan Content Flax Oil. Barlean's products are available nationwide in fine health food stores.*

**Barlean's Fishery**
4936 Lake Terrell Road
Ferndale, Washington 98248
Fax: (360) 384-1746
www.barleansfishery.com

*Interestingly, the same company that produces such great flax and other organic oils is known throughout the world for its wonderfully delicious and ecologically harvested wild salmon, which is so rich in marine omega-3 fatty acids. Their wild Pacific salmon is ecologically gathered from the waters of the Strait of Juan De Fuca, providing some of the purest wild salmon netted today. I love their canned smoked salmon, but they offer many different other varieties as well.*

**Brevail**

Lignan Research, LLC

9921 Carmel Mountain Road, #339

San Diego, California 92129

(888) 503-8300

www.brevail.com

Brevail *is an exciting and new self-care solution clinically tested to support breast and hormonal health. Women taking* Brevail *have reported improved mood and sense of well-being, and relief from symptoms associated with PMS and menopause.*

*If you don't consume lignan-rich flax daily, this is an essential supplement. (By the way, look for* Brevail *to soon introduce a men's lignan product for prostate health.)*

# References

1  Babu, U.S., et al. "Effect of dietary flaxseed on functions of peritoneal macrophages from young male and female rats." Experimental Biology 94, Parts I And II *Faseb Journal,* 1994.

2  Fernandes, G. & Venkatraman, J.T. "Role of omega-3 fatty acids in health and disease." *Nutr Res,* 1993; 13(suppl.1):S19-S45.

3  Taioli, E., et al. "Dietary habits and breast cancer: a comparative study of the United States and Italian data." *Nutrition and Cancer,* 1991; 16:259-265.

4  Ibid.

5  Yanagi, S., et al. "Sodium butryate inhibits the enhancing effect of high fat on mammary tumorigenesis." *Oncology,* 1993; 50(4):201-204.

6  Yam, D., et al. "Diet and disease—the Israeli paradox: possible dangers of a high omega-6 polyunsaturated fatty acid diet." *Israeli J Med Sci,*1996; 32:1134-1143.

7  Tham, D.M., et al. "Clinical review 97: Potential health benefits of dietary phytoestrogens: a review of the clinical, epidemiological, and mechanistic evidence." *J Clin Endocrinol Metab,* 1998; 83(7):2223-35.

8  Okuyama, H., et al. "Dietary fatty acids—the N-6 / N-3 balance and chronic elderly diseases. Excess linoleic acid and relative N-3 deficiency syndrome seen in Japan." *Prog Lipid Res,* 1997; 3(4):409-457.

9  Jeppesen, J., et al. "Triglyceride concentration and ischemic heart disease: an eight-year follow-up in the Copenhagen Male Study." *Circulation,* 1998; 97(11):1029-36.

10  Gotto, A.M. Jr. "Triglyceride: the forgotten risk factor." *Circulation,* 1998; 97(11):1027-8.

11  Associated Press. "Wider use seen for drugs to reduce cholesterol of heart patients." *The New York Times,* March 27, 1996: A1.

12  Ibid.

13  Newman, T.B. & Hully, S.B. "Carcinogenicity of lipid-lowering drugs." *Journal of the American Medical Association,* 1996; 275(1):55-60.

14  Associated Press. "Wider use seen for drugs to reduce cholesterol of heart patients." *The New York Times,* March 27, 1996: A1.

15  Hu, F.B., et al. "Dietary intake of alpha-linolenic acid and risk of fatal ischemic heart disease among women." *Am J Clin Nutr,* 1999; 69(5):890-897.

16  Sinclair, A.J., et al. "What is the role of alpha-linolenic acid for mammals?" *Lipids,* 2002; 37(12):1113-1123.

17  Baylin, A., et al. "Adipose tissue alpha-linolenic acid and nonfatal acute myocardial infarction in Costa Rica." *Circulation,* 2003;107(12):1586-1591.

18  de Lorgeril, M., et al. "Mediterranean diet, traditional risk factors, and the rate of cardiovascular complications after myocardial infarction. Final report of the Lyon Diet Heart Study." *Circulation*, 1999; 99:779-785.

19  Buajordet, I., et al. "Statins—the pattern of adverse effects with emphasis on mental reactions. Data from a national and an international database." *Tidsskr Nor Laegeforen*, 1997; 117:3210-3213.

20  Muldoon, M.F., et al. "Lowering cholesterol concentrations and mortality: A quantitative review of primary prevention trials." *BMJ*, 1990; 301:309-314.

21  Golomb, B.A. "Cholesterol and violence: Is there a connection?" *Ann Intern Med*, 1998; 128:478-487.

22  Harper, C.R. & Jacobson, T.A. "The fats of life: the role of omega-3 fatty acids in the prevention of coronary heart disease." *Arch Intern Med*, 2001; 161(18):2185-92.

23  Sandker, G.N., et al. "Serum cholesterol ester fatty acids and their relation with serum lipids in elderly men in Crete and the Netherlands." *Eur J Clin Nutr*, 1993; 47:201-208.

24  Kagawa, Y., et al. "Eicosapolyenlic acids of serum lipids of Japanese Islands with low incidence of cardiovascular diseases." *J Nutr Sci Vitaminol*, 1982; 28:441-453.

25  Prasad, K., et al. "Reduction of hypercholesterolemic atherosclerosis by CDC-flaxseed with very low alpha-linolenic acid." *Atherosclerosis*, 1998; 136(2):367-375.

26  Ferretti, A. & Flanagan, V.P. "Antithromboxane activity of dietary alpha-linolenic acid: a pilot study." *Prostaglandins Leukot Essent Fatty Acids*, 1996; 54(6):451-5.

27  Billman, G.E., et al. "Prevention of sudden cardiac death by dietary pure omega-3 polyunsaturated fatty acids in dogs." *Circulation*, 1999; 99(18):2452-2457.

28  Rallidis, L.S., et al. "Dietary alpha-linolenic acid decreases C-reactive protein, serum amyloid A and interleukin-6 in dyslipidaemic patients." *Atherosclerosis*, 2003; 167(2):237-242.

29  Ibid.

30  de Deckere, E.A., et al. "Health aspects of fish and n-3 polyunsaturated fatty acids from plant and marine origin." *Eur J Clin Nutr*, 1998; 52(10):749-53.

31  Kang, J.X. & Leaf, A. "Antiarrhythmic effects of polyunsaturated fatty acids: Recent studies." *Circulation*, 1996; 94:1774-1780.

32  Billman, G.E., et al. "Prevention of sudden cardiac death by dietary pure omega-3 polyunsaturated fatty acids in dogs." *Circulation*, 1999; 99(18):2452-2457.

33  Kang, J.X. & Leaf, A. "Protective effects of free polyunsaturated fatty acids on arrhythmias induced by lysophosphatidylcholine or palmitoylcarnitine in neonatal rat cardiac myocytes." *Eur J Pharmacol*, 1996; 297(1-2):97-106.

34  Billman, G.E., et al. "Prevention of sudden cardiac death by dietary pure omega-3 polyunsaturated fatty acids in dogs." *Circulation*, 1999; 99(18):2452-2457.

35   Kang, J.X. & Leaf, A. "Protective effects of free polyunsaturated fatty acids on arrhythmias induced by lysophosphatidylcholine or palmitoylcarnitine in neonatal rat cardiac myocytes." *Eur J Pharmacol*, 1996; 297(1-2):97-106.

36   Mori, T.A., et al. "Interactions between dietary fat, fish, and fish oils and their effects on platelet function in men at risk of cardiovascular disease." *Arterioscler Thromb Vasc Biol*, 1997; 17:279-286.

37   Enos, W.F., et al. "Coronary disease among United States soldiers killed in action in Korea." *J Amer Med Assoc*, 1953; 152(12):1090-1093.

38   Berry, E.M. & Hirsch, J. "Does dietary linolenic acid influence blood pressure?" *Am J Clin Nutr*, 1986; 44:336-340.

39   Ridker, P.M., et al. "Inflammation, aspirin, and the risk of cardiovascular disease in apparently healthy men." *N Eng J Med*, 1997; 336(14):973-979.

40   Fisher, M.K., et al. "Effects of dietary fish oil supplementation on polymorphonuclear leukocyte inflammatory potential." *Inflammation*, 1986; 10(4):387-92.

41   Dyerberg, J., et al. "Small is beautiful: alpha linolenic acid and eicosapentaenoic acid in man." *The Lancet*, May 21, 1983:1169.

42   Prasad, K. "Dietary flaxseed in prevention of hypercholesterolemic atherosclerosis." *Atherosclerosis*, 1997; 132(1):69-76.

43   Radack, K., et al. "Dietary supplementation with low-dose fish oils lowers fibrinogen levels: a randomized, double-blind controlled study." *Ann Int Med*, 1989; 11(9):757-758.

44   de Lorgeril, M., et al. "Mediterranean alpha-linolenic acid-rich diet in secondary prevention of coronary heart disease." *Lancet*, 1994; 343:1454-1459.

45   Hu, F.B., et al. "Dietary intake of alpha-linolenic acid and risk of fatal ischemic heart disease among women." *Am J Clin Nutr*, 1999; 69(5):890-897.

46   Shimokawa, T., et al. "Effect of dietary alpha-linolenate/linoleate balance on mean survival time, incidence of stroke and blood pressure of spontaneously hypertensive rats." *Life Sci*, 1988; 43:2067-2075.

47   Schmidt, E.B. & Dyerberg, J. "Omega-3 fatty acids. Current status in cardiovascular medicine." *Drugs*; 1994; 47:405-424.

48   Appel, L.J., et al. "Does supplementation of diet with 'fish oil' reduce blood pressure? A meta-analysis of controlled clinical trials." *Arch Intern Med*, 1993; 153:1429-1438.

49   Singer, P. "Alpha-linolenic acid vs. long-chain fatty acids in hypertension and hyperlipidemia." *Nutrition*, 1992; 8:133-135.

50   Chan, J.K., et al. "Dietary-alpha-linolenic acid is as effective as oleic acid and linoleic acid in lowering blood cholesterol in normolipidemic men." *Am J Clin Nutr*, 1991; 53:1230-1234.

51  Berry, E.M. & Hirsch, J. "Does dietary linolenic acid influence blood pressure?" *Am J Clin Nutr,* 1986; 44:336-340.

52  Ferretti, A. & Flanagan, V.P. "Antithromboxane activity of dietary alpha-linolenic acid: a pilot study." *Prostaglandins Leukot Essent Fatty Acids,* 1996; 54:451-455.

53  Trichopoulou, A., et al. "Consumption of olive oil and specific food groups in relation to breast cancer risk in Greece." *Journal of the National Cancer Institute,* 1995; 87(2):110-116.

54  Taioli, E., et al. "Dietary habits and breast cancer: a comparative study of the United States and Italian data." *Nutrition and Cancer,* 1991; 16:259-265.

55  Ibid.

56  Yanagi, S., et al. "Sodium butyrate inhibits the enhancing effect of high fat on mammary tumorigenesis." *Oncology,* 1993; 50(4):201-204.

57  Yam, D., et al. "Diet and disease—the Israeli paradox: possible dangers of a high omega-6 polyunsaturated fatty acid diet." *Israeli J Med Sci,* 1996; 32:1134-1143.

58  Thompson, L.U., et al. "Biological effects of dietary flaxseed in patients with breast cancer." *Breast Cancer Research and Treatment,* 2000; 64(1):50.

59  Thompson, L.U., et al. "Flaxseed and its lignan and oil components reduce mammary tumor growth at a late stage of carcinogenesis." *Carcinogenesis,* 1996; 17(6):1373-1376.

60  Rickard, S.E., et al. "Dose effects of flaxseed and its lignan on N-methyl-N-nitrosourea-induced mammary tumorigenesis in rats." *Nutr Cancer,* 1999; 35(1):50-57.

61  Orcheson, L.J., et al. "Flaxseed and its mammalian lignan precursor cause a lengthening or cessation of estrous cycling in rats." *Cancer Lett,* 1998; 125(1-2):69-76.

62  Tou, J.C. & Thompson, L.U. "Exposure to flaxseed or its lignan component during different developmental stages influences rat mammary gland structures." *Carcinogenesis,* 1999; 20(9):1831-1835.

63  Musey, P.I., et al. "Effect of diet on lignans and isoflavonoid phytoestrogens in chimpanzees." *Life Sci,* 1995; 57(7):655-664.

64  Pietinen, P., et al. "Serum enterolactone and risk of breast cancer: a case-control study in eastern Finland." *Cancer Epidemiol Biomarkers Prev,* 2000; 10(4):339-44.

65  Hutchins, A.M., et al. "Flaxseed consumption influences endogenous hormone concentrations in postmenopausal women." *Nutr Cancer,* 2001; 39(1):58-65.

66  Thompson, L.U., et al. "Biological effects of dietary flaxseed in patients with breast cancer." Abstract from the San Antonio Breast Cancer Symposium, December 2000.

67  Klein, V., et al. "Low alpha-linolenic acid content of adipose breast tissue is associated with an increased risk of breast cancer." *Eur J Cancer,* 2000; 36(3):335-40.

68  Bougnoux, P., et al. "Alpha-linolenic acid content of adipose breast tissue: a host determinant of the risk of early metastasis in breast cancer." *Br J Cancer,* 1994; 70:330-334.

69   Ingram, D., et al. "Case-control study of phyto-oestrogens and breast cancer." *Lancet,* 1997; 350(9083):990-994.

70   Chen, J. & Thompson, L.U. "Lignans and tamoxifen, alone or in combination, reduce human breast cancer cell adhesion, invasion and migration in vitro." *Breast Cancer Res Treat,* 2003; 80(2):163-170.

71   Horn-Ross, P.L., et al. "Phytoestrogen intake and endometrial cancer risk." *J Natl Cancer Inst,* 2003; 95(15):1158-1164.

72   Phipps, W.R., et al. "Effect of flax seed ingestion on the menstrual cycle." *J Clin Endocrinol Metab,* 1993; 77(5):1215-9.

73   Demark-Wahnefried, W., et al. "Pilot study of dietary fat restriction and flaxseed supplementation in men with prostate cancer before surgery: exploring the effects on hormonal levels, prostate-specific antigen, and histopathologic features." *Urology,* 2001; 58(1):47-52.

74   Denis, L., et al. "Diet and its preventive role in prostatic disease." *Eur Urol,* 1999; 35(5-6):377-387.

75   Yan, L., et al. "Dietary flaxseed supplementation and experimental metastasis of melanoma cells in mice." *Cancer Lett,* 1998; 124(2):181-186.

76   Sung, M.K., et al. "Mammalian lignans inhibit the growth of estrogen-independent human colon tumor cells." *Anticancer Res,* 1998; 18(3A):1405-1408.

77   Jenab, M. & Thompson, L.U. "The influence of flaxseed and lignans on colon carcinogenesis and beta-glucuronidase activity." *Carcinogenesis,* 1996; 17:1343-1348.

78   Falconer, J.S., et al. "Effect of eicosapentaenoic acid and other fatty acids on the growth in vitro of human pancreatic cancer cell lines." *Br J Cancer,* 1994; 69:826-832.

79   Simopoulos, A. *The Omega Plan.* New York: HarperCollins, 1999, pp. 86-98.

80   Rudin, D.O. & Felix, C. *Omega-3 Oils.* Honesdale, PA: Paragon Press, 1996, p. 216.

81   Hibbeln, J.R., et al. "Essential fatty acids predict metabolites of serotonin and dopamine in CSF among healthy controls, early and late onset alcoholics." *Biol Psychiatry,* 1998; 44:235-242.

82   Hibbeln, J.R., et al. "A replication study of violent and non-violent subjects: CSF metabolites of serotonin and dopamine are predicted by plasma essential fatty acids." *Biol Psychiatry,* 1998; 44:243-249.

83   Hibbeln, J.R. "Fish consumption and major depression." *Lancet,* 1998; 351:1213.

84   Mes, M., et al. "Fatty acid composition in major depression: Decreased omega-3 fractions in cholesteryl esters and increased C20:4 omega 6/C20:5 omega 3 ratio in cholesteryl esters and phospholipids." *J Affect Disord,* 1996; 38:35-46.

85   Adams, P.B., et al. "Arachadonic acid to eicosapentaneoic acid ratio in blood correlates positively with clinical symptoms of depression." *Lipids,* 1996; 31(suppl):S157-S161.

86  Edwards, R., et al. "Omega-3 polyunsaturated fatty acids in the diet and in the red blood cell membranes of depressed patients." *J Affect Disord,* 1998; 48:149-155.

87  Gitlin, M.J. & Pasnau, R.O. "Psychiatric syndromes linked to reproductive function in women: A review of current knowledge." *Am J Psychiatry,* 1989; 146(11):1413-1422.

88  Holman, R.T., et al. "Deficiency of essential fatty acids and membrane fluidity during pregnancy and lactation." *Proc Natl Acad Sci,* 1991; 88:4835-4839.

89  Ibid.

90  Virkkunen, M.E., et al. "Plasma phospholipid essential fatty acids and prostaglandins in alcoholic, habitually violent, and impulsive offenders." *Biological Psychiatry,* 1987; 22:1087-1096.

91  Kaplan, J.R., et al. "The effects of fat and cholesterol on social behavior in monkeys." *Psychosomatic Medicine,* 1991; 53:634-642.

92  Hamazaki, T.S., et al. "The effect of docosahexaenoic acid on aggression in young adults." *J of Clinical Investigation,* 1996; 97(4):1129-1134.

93  Hibbeln, J.R., et al. "A replication study of violent and non-violent subjects: CSF metabolites of serotonin and dopamine are predicted by plasma essential fatty acids." *Biol Psychiatry,* 1998; 44:243-249.

94  Singer, P. "Effects of dietary oleic, linoleic and alpha-linolenic acids on blood pressure, serum lipids, lipoproteins and the formation of eicosanoid precursors in patients with mild essential hypertension." *J of Human Hypertension,* 1990; 4:227-233.

95  Hibbeln, J.R. & Salem, N. "Dietary polyunsaturated fatty acids and depression: when cholesterol does not satisfy." *Amer J of Clin Nutr,* 1995; 62:1-9.

96  Hoffer, A. & Osmond, H. "Chronic schizophrenic patients treated ten years or more." *Journal of Orthomolecular Medicine,* 1993; 8:7-37.

97  Stoll, A.L. "Omega 3 fatty acids in bipolar disorder: a preliminary double-blind, placebo-controlled trial." *Arch Gen Psychiatry,* 1999; 56:407-412.

98  Holman, R.T., et al. "Deficiency of essential fatty acids and membrane fluidity during pregnancy and lactation." *Proc Natl Acad Sci,* 1991; 88:4835-4839.

99  Long, M. & Barrett, P. "Lawsuit is filed against Novartis on Ritalin sales." *The Wall Street Journal Europe,* May 15, 2000:4.

100  Adesman, A. "Does my child need Ritalin?" *Newsweek,* April 24, 2000:81.

101  Parker-Pope, T. "Drug firms research kids' one-a-day Ritalin." *The Wall Street Journal Europe,* May 15, 2000:31.

102  Rudin, D. & Felix, C. *Omega-3 Oils: A Practical Guide.* Garden City Park, NY: Avery Publishing, 1996.

103 Neuringer, M. & Conner, W.E. "N-3 fatty acids in the brain and retina: evidence for their essentiality." *Nutrition Reviews,* 1985; 44:285-294.

104 Tinoco, J. "Dietary requirement and function of alpha-linolenic acid in animals." *Prog. Lipid. Res,* 1982; 21:1-45.

105 Enslen, M., et al. "Effect of low intake of n-3 fatty acids during the development of brain phospholipid fatty acid composition and exploratory behavior in rats." *Lipids,* 1991; 26:203-208.

106 Reisbick, S., et al. "Home cage behavior of rhesus monkeys with long-term deficiency of omega-3 fatty acids." *Physiol Behav,* 1994; 55:231-239.

107 Colquhoun, I. & Bunday, S. "A lack of essential fatty acids as a possible cause of hyperactivity in children." *Med Hypotheses,* 1981; 7:673-679.

108 Mitchell, E.A., et al. "Essential fatty acids and maladjusted behaviour in children." *Prostaglandins Leukot Med,* 1983; 12(3):281-7.

109 Mitchell, E., et al. "Clinical characteristics and serum essential fatty acid levels in hyperactive children." *Clin Pediatr,* 1987; 26:406-411.

110 Stevens, L., et al. "Essential fatty acid metabolism in boys with attention-deficit hyperactivity disorder." *American Journal of Clinical Nutrition,* 1995; 62:761-8.

111 Stevens, L., et al. "Omega-3 fatty acids in boys with behavior, learning, and health problems." *Physiology & Behavior,* 1996; 59(4-5):915-20.

112 Bekaroğlu, M., et al. "Relationships between serum free fatty acids and zinc, and attention deficit hyperactivity disorder: a research note." *J Child Psychol Psychiatry,* 1996; 37(2):225-227.

113 *Developmental Medicine & Child Neurology,* 2000; 42:174-181.

114 Burkitt, D. & Trowell, H. *Western Diseases: Their Emergence and Prevention.* Cambridge, MA: Harvard University Press, 1981.

115 Vessby, B., et al. "The risk to develop NIDDM is related to the fatty acid composition of the serum cholesterol esters." *Diabetes,* 1994; 43(11):1353-7.

116 Hainault, I.M., et al. "Fish oil in a high lard diet prevents obesity, hyperlipidemia, and adipocyte insulin resistance in rats." *Annals of New York Academy of Sciences,* 1993; 683:98-101.

117 Ikemoto, S., et al. "High-fat diet-induced hyperglycemia and obesity in mice: Differential effects of dietary oils." *Metabolism,* 1996; 45(12):1539-1546.

118 Storlien, L.H. "Skeletal muscle membrane lipids and insulin resistance." *Lipids,* 1996; 31(Supplement):S-261-265.

119 Torjesen, P.A., et al. "Lifestyle changes may reverse development of the insulin resistance syndrome." *Diabetes Care,* 1997; 30:26-31.

120 Fanaian, M., et al. "The effect of modified fat diet on insulin resistance and metabolic parameters in type 2 diabetes." *Diabetologia,* 1996; 39(1):A7.

121  Murray, M. & Pizzorno, J. *Encyclopedia of Natural Medicine.* Rocklin, CA: Prima Publishing, 1998:448-454, 763-769.

122  Ziboh, V.A. "Implications of dietary oils and polyunsaturated fatty acids in the management of cutaneous disorders." *Arch Dermatol,* 1989; 125(2):241-5.

123  Kruger, M.C. & Horrobin, D.F. "Calcium metabolism, osteoporosis and essential fatty acids: a review." *Prog Lipid Res,* 1997; 36(2-3):131-151.

124  Schlemmer, C.K., et al. "Oestrogen and essential fatty acid supplementation corrects bone loss due to ovariectomy in the female Sprague Dawley rat." *Prostaglandins Leukot Essent Fatty Acids,* 1999; 61(6):381-390.

125  Schlemmer, C.K., et al. "Ectopic calcification of rat aortas and kidneys is reduced with n-3 fatty acid supplementation." *Prostaglandins Leukot Essent Fatty Acids,* 1998; 59(3):221-227.

126  Kruger, M.C., et al. "Calcium, gamma-linolenic acid and eicosapentaenoic acid supplementation in senile osteoporosis." *Aging (Milano),* 1998; 10(5):385-394.

127  De Leo, V., et al. "Polycystic ovary syndrome and type 2 diabetes mellitus." *Minerva Ginecol,* 2004; 56(1):53-62.

128  Pelusi, B., et al. "Type 2 diabetes and the polycystic ovary syndrome." *Minerva Ginecol,* 2004; 56(1):41-51.

129  Norman, R.J., et al. "Polycystic ovary syndrome." *Med J Aust,* 2004; 180(3):132-7.

130  Ikemoto, S., et al. "High-fat diet-induced hyperglycemia and obesity in mice: Differential effects of dietary oils." *Metabolism,* 1996; 45(12):1539-1546.

131  Lemay, A., et al. "Flaxseed dietary supplement versus hormone replacement therapy in hypercholesterolemic menopausal women." *Obstet Gynecol,* 2002; 100(3):495-504.

132  Hainault, I.M., et al. "Fish oil in a high lard diet prevents obesity, hyperlipidemia, and adipocyte insulin resistance in rats." *Annals of New York Academy of Sciences,* 1993; 683:98-101.

133  Storlien, L.H. "Skeletal muscle membrane lipids and insulin resistance." *Lipids,* 1996; 31(Supplement):S-261-265.

134  Yam, D., et al. "Diet and disease—the Israeli paradox; possible dangers of a high omega-6 polyunsaturated fatty acid diet." *Isr J Med Sci,* 1996; 32:1134-1143.

135  Torjesen, P.A., et al. "Lifestyle changes may reverse development of the insulin resistance syndrome." *Diabetes Care,* 1997; 30:26-31.

136  Fanaian, M., et al. "The effect of modified fat diet on insulin resistance and metabolic parameters in type 2 diabetes." *Diabetologia,* 1996; 39(1):A7.

137  Kelso, K.A., et al. "Effects of dietary supplementation with alpha-linolenic acid on the phospholipid fatty acid composition and quality of spermatozoa in cockerel from 24 to 72 weeks of age." *J Reprod Fertil,* 1997 May; 110(1):53-59.

138 Christophe, A., et al. "Intake of Alpha Linolenic Acid, but not of Docosahexaenoic Acid, correlates positively with DHA content, and with parameters for fertilization potential of human spermatozoa." Abstract for 90th AOCS Annual Meeting. Orlando, Florida: 1999.

139 Attar-Bashi, N.M., et al. "Alpha-linolenic acid and the risk of prostate cancer. What is the evidence?" *J Urol*, 2004; 171(4):1402-7.

140 Kolonel, L.N., et al. "Dietary fat and prostate cancer: current status." *J Natl Cancer Inst*, 1999; 91(5):414-28.

141 Harvei, S., et al. "Prediagnostic level of fatty acids in serum phospholipids: omega-3 and omega-6 fatty acids and the risk of prostate cancer." *Int J Cancer*, 1997; 71(4):545-51.

142 Godley, P.A., et al. "Biomarkers of essential fatty acid consumption and risk of prostatic carcinoma." *Cancer Epidemiol Biomarkers Prev*, 1996; 5(11):889-95.

143 Giovannucci, E., et al. "A prospective study of dietary fat and risk of prostate cancer." *J Natl Cancer Inst*, 1993; 85(19):1571-9.

144 Gann, P.H., et al. "Prospective study of plasma fatty acids and risk of prostate cancer." *J Natl Cancer Inst*, 1994; 86(4):281-6.

145 Andersson, S.O., et al. "Energy, nutrient intake and prostate cancer risk: a population-based case-control study in Sweden." *Int J Cancer*, 1996; 68(6):716-22.

146 Mori, M., et al. "A review of cohort studies on the association between history of diabetes mellitus and occurrence of cancer." *Asian Pac J Cancer Prev*, 2000; 1(4):269-276.

147 Rickard, S.E., et al. "Plasma insulin-like growth factor I levels in rats are reduced by dietary supplementation of flaxseed or its lignan secoisolariciresinol diglycoside." *Cancer Lett*, 2000; 161(1):47-55.

148 Chen, J., et al. "Dietary flaxseed inhibits human breast cancer growth and metastasis and downregulates expression of insulin-like growth factor and epidermal growth factor receptor." *Nutr Cancer*, 2002; 43(2):187-192.

149 Dabrosin, C., et al. "Flaxseed inhibits metastasis and decreases extracellular vascular endothelial growth factor in human breast cancer xenografts." *Cancer Lett*, 2002; 185(1):31-37.

150 Shapiro, J.A., et al. "Diet and rheumatoid arthritis in women: a possible protective effect of fish consumption." *Epidemiology*, 1996; 7(3):256-63.

151 Kremer, J.M., et al. "Effects of high-dose fish oil on rheumatoid arthritis after stopping nonsteroidal antiinflammatory drugs. Clinical and immune correlates." *Arthritis and Rheumatism*, 1995; 38(8):1107-14.

152 Lau, C.S., et al. "Effects of fish oil on plasma fibrinolysis in patients with mild rheumatoid arthritis." *Clinical and Experimental Rheumatology*, 1995; 13(1):87-90.

153 Lozano, P., et al. "The economic burden of asthma in US children: estimates from the National Medical Expenditure Survey." *J Allergy Clin Immunol*, 1999; 104(5):957-963.

154 Clark, N.M., et al. "Childhood asthma." *Environ Health Perspect,* 1999; 107 Suppl 3:421-429.

155 Weiler, J.M. & Ryan, E.J. 3rd. "Asthma in United States olympic athletes who participated in the 1998 olympic winter games." *J Allergy Clin Immunol,* 2000; 106(2):267-271.

156 Broughton, K.S., et al. "Reduced asthma symptoms with n-3 fatty acid ingestion are related to 5-series leukotriene production." *Am J Clin Nutr,* 1997; 65:1011-1017.

157 Hodge, L., et al. "Consumption of oily fish and childhood asthma risk." *MJA,* 1996; 164:137-140.

158 Okamoto, M., et al. "Effects of perilla seed oil supplementation on leukotriene generation by leucocytes in patients with asthma associated with lipometabolism." *International Archives of Allergy and Immunology,* 2000; 122(2):137-142.

159 Okamoto, M., et al. "Effects of dietary supplementation with n-3 fatty acids compared with n-6 fatty acids on bronchial asthma." *Intern Med,* 2000; 39(2):107-111.

160 Hashimoto, N., et al. "[Effects of eicosapentaenoic acid in patients with bronchial asthma]." *Nihon Kyobu Shikkan Gakkai Zasshi,* 1997; 35(6):634-640.

161 Cameron, J.S. "Lupus nephritis: an historical perspective 1968-1998." *J Nephrol,* 1999; 12 Suppl 2:S29-41.

162 Velasquez, M.T. & Bhathena, S.J. "Dietary phytoestrogens: a possible role in renal disease protection." *Am J Kidney Dis,* 2001; 37(5):1056-1068.

163 Clark, W.F., et al. "A novel treatment for lupus nephritis: lignan precursor derived from flax." *Lupus* 2000; 9(6):429-436.

164 Hall, A.V., et al. "Abrogation of MRL/lpr lupus nephritis by dietary flaxseed." *Am J Kidney Dis,* 1993; 22(2):326-332.

165 Ogborn, M.R., et al. "Flaxseed ameliorates interstitial nephritis in rat polycystic kidney disease." *Kidney Int,* 1999; 55(2):417-23.

166 Clark, W.F. "Flaxseed in lupus nephritis: a two-year nonplacebo-controlled crossover study." *J Am Coll Nutr,* 2001; 20(2 Suppl):143-148.

167 Li, D., et al. "Relationship between platelet phospholipid FA and mean platelet volume in healthy men." *Lipids,* 2002; 37(9):901-6.

168 Krajcovicová-Kudláčková, M., et al. "Plasma fatty acid profile and alternative nutrition." *Ann Nutr Metab,* 1997; 41(6):365-370.

169 Li, D., et al. "Effect of dietary alpha-linolenic acid on thrombotic risk factors in vegetarian men." *Am J Clin Nutr,* 1999; 69(5):872-882.

170 Sanders, T.A., et al. "Essential fatty acid requirements of vegetarians in pregnancy, lactation, and infancy." *Am J Clin Nutr,* 1999; 70(3 Suppl):555S-559S.

# Index

# About the Author

Herb Joiner-Bey, N.D., is an experienced primary-care natural health practitioner, specializing in classical homeopathy, therapeutic nutrition, Western botanical medicine, and the conventional treatment of sexually transmitted diseases. He places strong focus on emotional, social, and spiritual aspects of healing. He is also a dynamic professional educator and seminar leader who has trained thousands of health care professionals in the philosophy and clinical application of modern, scientifically verified natural medicine. Dr. Bey is the author of several books, a CD-ROM, and numerous articles in this field. In addition, he serves as medical/scientific editor for several journals and magazines focused on integrative medicine. He is an adjunct professor of classical homeopathy and advanced therapeutics at Bastyr University, Kenmore, Washington, and a consultant to several manufacturers of the highest-quality products in the nutriceutical/health food industry, including Barlean's Organic Oils. He also serves as guest speaker on natural medicine for radio talk shows across the nation. Dr. Bey holds a B.A. degree in physics from Johns Hopkins University, Baltimore, Maryland, and an N.D. (Doctor of Naturopathic Medicine) degree from Bastyr University.